So you're having a

Hysterectomy

Includes Alternatives to Hysterectomy

So you're having a

Hysterectomy

TOGAS TULANDI MD
BARBARA LEVY MD

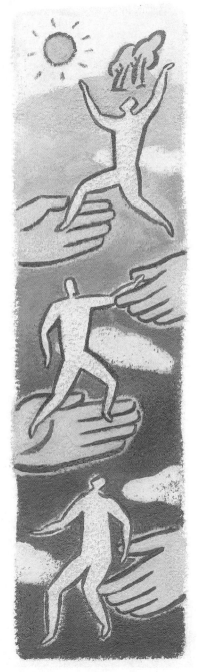

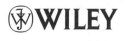 WILEY

Published by John Wiley & Sons, Inc., 111 River Street, Hoboken, NJ 07030

First published in Canada in a somewhat different form by SCRIPT Medical Press, Inc. in 2003.
Copyright © 2003 SCRIPT Medical Press, Inc.

Library of Congress Cataloging-in-Publication Data

Tulandi, T. (Togas)
  So you're having a hysterectomy / Togas Tulandi, Barbara Levy.
      p. cm.
Includes index.
  ISBN 0-470-83345-9 (Paper)
  1. Hysterectomy—Popular works. 2. Patient education. I. Levy, Barbara S. II. Title.
RG391 .T84 2003
618.1'453—dc22

                              2003020790

Series Creator: Helen Byrt
Senior Editor: Jenny Lass
Copy Editor: Andrea Knight
Series Design: Rocket Design
Typesetting: Angela Bobotsis
Cover Illustration: Ross Paul Lindo
Author Photograph: Pierre Dubois, Medical Multimedia Services, McGill University Health Centre
Book Illustrations: Zane Waldman
Publishing Consultant: Malcolm Lester & Associates

Photograph on page 88 courtesy of the Audio-Visual Department, Sir Mortimer B. Davis Jewish General Hospital, Montréal. The material on pages 67-68 and 159-161 first appeared in *So You're Having Angioplasty—What Happens Next?* by Stephen Fort MD and Victoria Foulger RN, published by SCRIPT Medical Press in 2001. This material appears here by courtesy of the authors.

The publisher has made every effort to obtain permissions for use of copyrighted material in this book; any errors or omissions will be corrected in the next printing.

Printed and bound in Canada
10 9 8 7 6 5 4 3 2 1

To my family and my patients

———

T.T.

To my patients, who have taught me more than textbooks
ever could, about women and women's health

———

B.L.

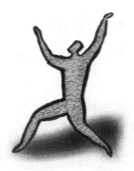

acknowledgments

The publisher's particular thanks go to Rosane Reis for allowing the twinkle in our eye to become a reality. *What Happens Next?* veterans Dr. Stuart McCluskey and Victoria Foulger RN once again shared their expertise for the sections on anesthetics/blood conservation, and herbal medicines, respectively, and Dr. Stephen Holzapfel taught us about the needs of partners. Thanks are also due to the talented creative team who never flagged in their enthusiasm: Angela Bobotsis, Jenny Lass, Andrea Knight, Zane Waldman, Sarah Ternoway, Malcolm Lester, and Debra Beck.

Finally, our gratitude and admiration are extended to all the marvelous women who allowed us to share their experiences, good, bad, painful, and personal. We can't name you here, but you know who you are. You give this book its soul. Thank you.

disclaimer

THE INFORMATION PROVIDED IN THIS BOOK MAY NOT
apply to all patients, all clinical situations, all hospitals,
or all eventualities, and is not intended to be a
substitute for the advice of a qualified physician or other
medical professional. Always consult a qualified physician
about anything that affects your health, especially before
starting an exercise program or using a complementary
therapy not prescribed by your doctor.

The publisher and the authors make no representations or
warranties with respect to the accuracy or completeness of the
contents of this work and specifically disclaim all warranties,
including without limitation any implied warranties of fitness
for a particular purpose. No warranty may be created or
extended by any promotional statements. Neither the
publisher nor the authors shall be liable for any damages
arising herefrom.

contents

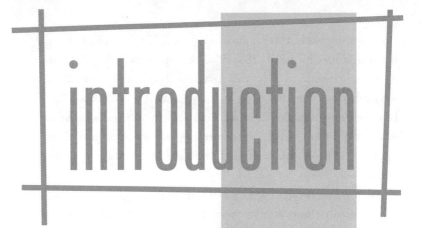

introduction

If you have been told that you need a hysterectomy or surgical removal of the uterus, you are in good company. Hysterectomy is the second most common surgical procedure performed in North America (after cesarean section), with about 600,000 hysterectomies performed each year in the United States and about 60,000 in Canada. Twenty to 30 percent of all hysterectomies are done for excessive uterine bleeding, even though in some cases the uterus itself is anatomically normal. Inevitably, many women (and men) have started asking whether all these procedures are really necessary.

You are the most important part of your health care team and only you can decide what treatment you want. While in some cases hysterectomy is life saving, and in many others it is life changing—for the better—it is also true that too many hysterectomies in the past were performed without women being aware of alternatives to control their symptoms. This book aims to help you decide whether hysterectomy is the best choice for you. Hysterectomy is often the right answer, but it should no longer be viewed as the answer to every gynecological problem. There are now many excellent alternatives to hysterectomy and Chapter 7 covers these in detail.

Hysterectomy itself can be performed by different routes, including through the vagina or by means of a small telescope through the belly-button, and Chapter 6 covers all the options. Chapter 3 brings all these choices together to help you decide between them, by discussing whether hysterectomy is right for you, and if so, what kind of hysterectomy you need. Chapter 2 walks you through the ladder of tests you should have before determining that hysterectomy is needed, and Chapter 11 gives you some benchmarks to decide if your procedure was successful.

After a hysterectomy, especially if you have your ovaries removed and are suddenly thrown into menopause, there are many adjustments to be made, but the good news is that there is also a host of things that you can do to take control and change your life for the better. In Chapter 10 we share some practical advice for everything from diet to sexual difficulties, as well as step-by-step instruction on important techniques such as breast exams and pelvic floor exercises.

If you need a refresher on how your uterus and other reproductive organs work, Chapter 1 provides the answers, and Chapter 12 will walk you through the maze of hormone replacement therapy. Finally, Chapter 13 gives a sample of upcoming technologies and techniques that are being developed to help women in the future.

This book is not designed to replace your discussions with your doctor, but to add to them. Our goal is to provide you and your family with enough information to understand why your physician is advising a particular course of action, and to give you the confidence to request a second opinion if you don't agree with that advice. In essence, our hope is that this book will give you the power to take control of your future and be happy with the choices that you make.

Good luck!

—Togas Tulandi, MD
—Barbara Levy, MD

Chapter

you and your uterus

What Happens in this Chapter

- The facts on your vagina, uterus, cervix and ovaries
- Their roles in both reproduction and sex
- What do your hormones do?
- How it all works together
- What can go wrong

Your uterus is one part of a complicated and remarkable piece of machinery: your reproductive organs. Your internal and external reproductive organs play different roles in sex and reproduction, directed by the rise and fall of hormones. When things start to go wrong, most women experience the same symptoms in varying degrees—heavy bleeding and/or pelvic pain. There are many different causes for these symptoms, but be assured that most of them are not life threatening. This chapter takes you through the basics of how your reproductive system works, and what happens when it doesn't.

What Are Reproductive Organs For?

THE ANSWER TO THIS QUESTION MAY APPEAR PRETTY OBVIOUS—reproductive organs are for reproduction—but if it were that simple, this book would be half as long as it is. Your reproductive organs have many potential roles. They define you as female, they can give you pleasure during sex, they produce hormones that keep you healthy—and they help make babies. The point is, because reproductive organs mean so many different things in different ways to different people, a procedure to remove them is bound to generate debate. A woman (or gynecologist) who believes that a uterus is just for babies, and the woman has all the babies she wants, will have no problem with hysterectomy. On the other hand, a woman who believes that an intact uterus is essential for a good sex life will strongly resist a total hysterectomy. In order to understand hysterectomy fully, and the alternatives, there is only one place to start: with a frank discussion about your reproductive organs and what they do.

External Reproductive Organs

The Vulva

The external sex organs of women are shown in Figure I–I. The correct name for this part of the body is the **vulva**. If you hold a mirror between your legs, everything you can see apart from your anus is the vulva. In the center of the vulva is the opening of the **vagina**, and above it, the opening of the urinary tract or **urethra**. The **hymen** is a thin membrane that stretches across the opening of the vagina in some women. An intact hymen theoretically indicates that a woman is a virgin; however, this is not always true: the hymen can be torn by many activities other than sex, such as gymnastics, and the hymen can remain intact even after intercourse.

At the top of the vulva, just below the pubic bone, is the **clitoris** (Greek word for "key"). The clitoris is equivalent to the penis in men, and consists of a small shaft and a tip, or **glans**, that projects outward covered by a hood of skin. Just like the penis, the clitoris has thousands of nerve endings, making it extremely sensitive to stimulation. It also becomes swollen and erect during sexual excitement.

Not surprisingly, all these delicate structures need protection, and this is the role of the two sets of **labia** (or lips) that surround the vulva on both sides and meet at the top, above the clitoris.

If you have undergone genital mutilation or **female circumcision**, your vulva will not look like this.

Reproductive Role

The vulva has no specific role in reproduction, apart from encouraging reproduction by making sex pleasurable.

Sexual Role

As the "pleasure center" of the body, the vulva has a central role in a woman's sexual experience. Although a woman can receive sexual enjoyment by stimulation of many parts of her body, it is generally accepted that the clitoris is the major organ involved in sexual excitement. Studies have shown that the clitoris is also the primary source of all orgasms, whether these are experienced as "vaginal" or "clitoral"—the physical response is the same. Recent studies of the anatomy of the clitoris may explain why this is. It was previously thought that the clitoris was just the small organ visible on the outside of the body, but anatomical studies have shown that the clitoris extends further back into the body. While it's still not certain how all the different sensations experienced during sex work together to produce an orgasm, the clitoris clearly has a central role. This makes sense, since the clitoris is equivalent to a man's penis. This is important information when considering hysterectomy, since there will be no alteration in the vulva or the function of the clitoris with any form of hysterectomy.

Figure 1–1. The Vulva

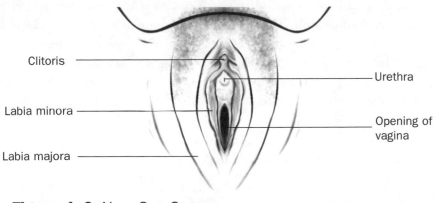

Clitoris

Labia minora

Labia majora

Urethra

Opening of vagina

Figure 1–2. Your Sex Organs

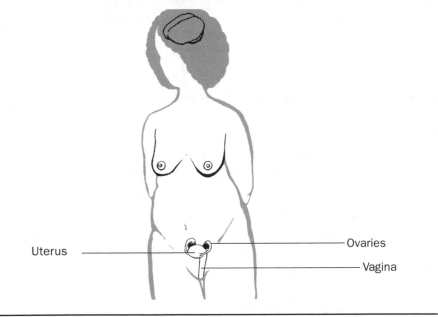

Uterus

Ovaries

Vagina

Although the uterus and ovaries are the main organs of reproduction, other areas, such as the brain and breasts, are also important to your sexual experience.

The Breasts

Although not strictly speaking reproductive organs, the breasts have a role in both reproduction, by producing milk for the new baby, and sex, as sexual attractants and erogenous zones (see Figure 1–2).

Internal Reproductive Organs

The Vagina

The vagina is a muscular tube about 8 cm (3 inches) long that leads to the uterus and can stretch as needed for sexual intercourse or childbirth. Although we think of the vagina as being "inside" you, in fact, like your mouth, it is constantly exposed to the outside world (for instance during bathing or intercourse), so it must have good defenses. It therefore has a tough inner lining to avoid damage and secretes slightly acidic fluid, that discourages infection. The thick vaginal walls and the acid secretions are encouraged by the

---

Vaginal Lubrication **[MORE DETAIL]**

The vagina is kept clean and moist partly by mucous secretions from the cervix. These secretions vary from almost clear around ovulation to milky white after ovulation. Vaginal lubrication during sexual excitement comes from several different places:

- **Bartholin's glands** – These glands produce a clear fluid that comes out between the hymen and the labia minora (see Figure 1–1)
- **Skene's glands** – The secretion from these glands comes out around the urethral opening. These glands are thought to be responsible for the fluid "ejaculation" experienced by some women at orgasm.
- **Vaginal walls** – During sexual arousal, there is greatly increased blood flow to the walls of the vagina which increases its length by about 30 percent. As a result, fluid seeps through the walls of the vagina into the passageway. Decreased blood flow to the vagina due to smoking or diabetes, or low estrogen, can therefore lead to painful sex.

presence of estrogen. This is one of the reasons why women are more prone to vaginal infections and discomfort after menopause, when estrogen levels fall. Vaginal lubrication also diminishes after menopause (see More Detail box on page 5).

Reproductive Role

The role of the vagina in reproduction is to provide a passage for sperm into the body and a passage for a baby out of the body. During childbirth the vagina is called the **birth canal**.

Sexual Role

The vagina has fewer nerve endings than the vulva (especially the clitoris) and is not very sensitive to sexual stimulation. Because the vagina is supplied with nerves from the whole pelvic area, it is difficult from a medical point of view to pinpoint exactly where pleasure arises. In 1950 a German physician named Grafenberg described an erogenous pressure-point called the **G-spot** about halfway up the vagina on the front wall. Although anatomical studies haven't located a definite structure here, one suggestion is that the sensitivity of the G-spot (if any) may be due to the underlying Skene's glands (see page 5), the equivalent of the prostate gland in men.

The muscles that support the vagina can sag as a result of childbirth or the aging process, diminishing sexual pleasure for both partners. **Kegel exercises** (see page 168) can correct this problem.

The Uterus

The **uterus (womb)** is a muscular, hollow organ approximately the size and shape of an upside-down pear. The upper part of the uterus is called the **body** and the long, narrow neck that connects the body to the vagina is called the **cervix** (see Figure 1–3). The cervix sticks out into the vagina, so it can be felt from inside the vagina as a firm projection. The space inside the uterus is triangular and lined with a unique layer, called the **endometrium**, which in turn is surrounded by a thick muscle layer (the **myometrium**).

Figure 1–3. Internal Sex Organs

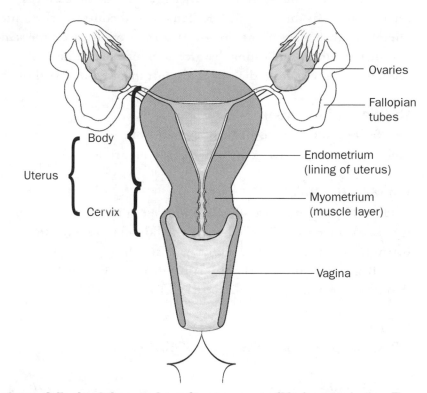

The uterus, fallopian tubes, and ovaries are responsible for reproduction. The ovaries also produce several important hormones. The vagina plays a role in both sexual function and reproduction.

Reproductive Role

The uterus is the place where the fertilized egg is implanted and grows into a baby over a period of 9 months. Every month, the endometrium becomes thick in preparation for the arrival and implantation of a fertilized egg. If pregnancy does not occur, the top layer of the endometrium dies and is shed during **menstruation**.

Sexual Role

The sexual role of the uterus is unclear. Although the uterus expands and lifts during sexual excitement and contracts rhythmically during orgasm, many women report that their orgasms are the same after hysterectomy, indicating that, for a significant number of women, sensations from the uterus are not involved in sexual pleasure.

The Fallopian Tubes

The **fallopian tubes** are a pair of curved hollow tubes that run from each side of the uterus to the ovaries (see Figure 1–3).

Reproductive Role

The fallopian tubes are the place where egg meets sperm. The new egg leaves the ovary, is picked up by the fallopian tube, is fertilized (or not), and then enters the uterus. If fertilized, the egg will then grow into a baby or, if it is not fertilized, it will be expelled during the next menstrual period or absorbed by the body.

Sexual Role

The fallopian tubes do not have a role in sex.

The Ovaries

The **ovaries** are roughly the size and shape of a small chicken egg and are located at the end of each fallopian tube. Each ovary is a bundle of thousands of small sacs called **follicles**, each of which contains an egg.

Reproductive Role

Ovaries are the key reproductive organs in women, equivalent to the testes in men. At birth, the ovary contains about half a million eggs. By puberty there are 300,000 or less, but this is more than enough for one egg to be released per menstrual cycle for the next

30 to 40 years. The ovaries also secrete sex hormones. For more on the role of ovaries, see later in this chapter.

Sexual Role

The ovaries' role in sex is unclear. If they have any involvement, it is indirect, by secreting the hormones estrogen, progesterone and testosterone. In many mammals these hormones control the mating urge (**heat**). In humans, only testosterone appears to have a direct role in sexual desire.

The Brain

It has been said that the brain is the most important sex organ of all. A woman's attitude to sex, to herself, to her partner, and her day-to-day mood can have a powerful effect on sexual interest. Other psychological influences such as imagination and past experiences can also help or hinder sexual enjoyment. This new understanding of the role of the brain in both good sex and bad sex is what allows sex therapy to be effective for many people.

The brain is also important in the reproductive process because it controls the rise and fall of the sex hormones.

Hormones

The main hormones involved in sex and reproduction are **estrogen, progesterone, testosterone, follicle-stimulating hormone (FSH)**, and **luteinizing hormone (LH)**. Estrogen is possibly the most familiar of these hormones but the others all have important supporting roles to play.

Estrogen

Estrogen has hundreds of complicated roles, but basically it stimulates growth. There are three different kinds: **estrone** (or **E1**),

The Many Faces of Estrogen

What estrogen (estradiol) does	What this means	
	Before menopause	After menopause
Promotes the growth and maintenance of the uterus and vagina	• Reproductive organs develop at puberty • Vagina is thick, flexible and well lubricated • Endometrium (womb lining) grows each month	• Uterus shrinks (slightly) • Vagina is dryer and more prone to damage • Pregnancy is not possible in normal circumstances
Promotes growth and maintenance of secondary sex characteristics	• "Womanly" shape develops • Breasts stay healthy and capable of producing milk	• Breasts change in appearance
Controls brain hormones by "feedback loop"	• Menstrual cycle is regulated	• Menstrual cycles cease
Promotes bone health	• Bones stay strong and healthy	• Bones become weaker and more porous • Risk of osteoporosis increases
Maintains healthy blood vessels	• Women's risk of heart disease is lower than men's	• Risk of heart disease increases and becomes the same as for men

What estrogen (estradiol) does	What this means	
	Before menopause	After menopause
Maintains healthy skin	• Skin is firm, flexible and well moisturized	• Skin is thinner and drier
Causes fat to accumulate under the skin, especially on the thighs, breasts and buttocks	• Female "curvy" shape is maintained • Fat stores develop that are useful for energy during pregnancy and breastfeeding.	• Uncertain: many women put on weight *more* easily after menopause, and in different places, for example around the stomach.
May help to maintain healthy brain cells	• Possibly: cognitive function (memory and thinking ability) declines more slowly with age.	• Uncertain: studies disagree about whether estrogen therapy after menopause can prevent diseases such as Alzheimer's.
Increases sexual desire in many animals	• No direct role in human females, but has an indirect role by maintaining vaginal blood flow and lubrication thus encouraging arousal and pain-free penetration.	• Lack of estrogen does not affect sexual desire directly, but a drier vagina may make sex less enjoyable and appealing.
Affects emotions?	• Science has not been able to prove or disprove that estrogen affects mood. In most women physical symptoms (e.g., menstrual discomfort) and psychological factors are probably much more important than estrogen levels.	• Estrogen replacement therapy's "magical" effect on mood probably has more to do with relieving uncomfortable symptoms than with a direct effect on emotions.
Controls sleep problems	• Healthy sleep patterns	• More sleep problems, for example, frequent night waking.

estradiol (E2), and **estriol** (E3). Although we generally refer to "estrogen" in this book to keep things simple, it is sometimes useful to know about these different types.

Estrone is the "inactive" form of estrogen and the main estrogen you will produce after menopause. It is made by your ovaries before menopause and by your body fat after menopause. Estradiol is the "active" form of estrogen and the star of the show before menopause. It is produced by the ovaries. Some of the effects of estradiol in the body are summarized on pages 10 and 11.

Estriol is the least potent type of estrogen and is only produced by the placenta of pregnant women.

Progesterone

Progesterone is the most important sex hormone after estrogen. The ovaries start to produce progesterone in large quantities during the second half of the menstrual cycle. The role of progesterone is to prepare the body for a fertilized egg, or pregnancy—thus its name: **pro**(moting) **gest**(ation). Progesterone maintains the lining of the uterus, allowing it to grow thick and spongy. Progesterone is also responsible for the sweet cravings, sluggish digestion, bloated feeling, breast tenderness, and fatigue that many women experience as their periods approach. This may be the body maximizing its energy intake in preparation for pregnancy.

Testosterone

Testosterone is thought of as a male hormone, but women also produce it. It is one of a group of hormones called **androgens**. Before menopause, estrogen is more dominant than testosterone, but as estrogen levels decrease at menopause, testosterone can temporarily take over. This explains why some older women start to grow coarse facial hair. Testosterone's helpful effects include sexual desire, muscle and bone strength, and increased energy. Fat tissue can convert testosterone to estrogen, so overweight women tend to have more bleeding problems due to excess estrogen.

Brain Hormones

The sex hormones produced by the **pituitary gland**, which sits directly under the brain, are follicle stimulating hormone (FSH), which makes an egg ripen, and luteinizing hormone (LH), which causes the egg to be released. FSH and LH are indirectly controlled by levels of estrogen and progesterone, and are under the direct control of a brain hormone called **gonadotrophin-releasing hormone**.

How It All Works Together

The amazingly complicated changes in a woman's body over the course of her life—puberty, the menstrual cycle, childbirth, menopause—generally happen automatically as the sex hormones rise and fall on cue, controlled by the brain and each other. Before looking at what can go wrong, it's worth looking at what happens when it all goes right. We will concentrate on the menstrual cycle and menopause. Puberty and pregnancy are outside the scope of this book.

The Menstrual Cycle

The purpose of the menstrual cycle is to produce a new egg each month for fertilization. If the egg is not fertilized, it is passed out of the body and a new cycle begins.

Day 1 of the cycle is the first day of your menstrual period. The cycle starts when the pituitary gland releases FSH (see Figure 1–4). The follicles in the ovary start to secrete estrogen and one follicle starts to ripen. Estrogen levels in the body gradually increase and trigger other changes, such as growth of the lining of the uterus.

Around Day 12, the high levels of estrogen stimulate the pituitary gland to produce LH. This is the turning-point of the cycle. The sudden surge of LH triggers **ovulation**, when the ripened follicle suddenly ruptures and releases the egg. Ovulation happens around Day 14. The egg must be fertilized in the next 36 hours or it will die.

As the egg moves down one of the fallopian tubes, the follicle it leaves behind starts producing progesterone in large quantities. Progesterone levels now rise. Over the next 14 days, estrogen and progesterone prepare the lining of the uterus for the fertilized egg.

If the egg is not fertilized, and pregnancy does not occur, the estrogen and progesterone levels fall right back to their starting point. The wall of the uterus, no longer supported by the hormones, is shed. This process, only too familiar to the vast majority of women, is called **menstruation** or **menses**.

Figure 1–4. Hormone Levels in the Menstrual Cycle

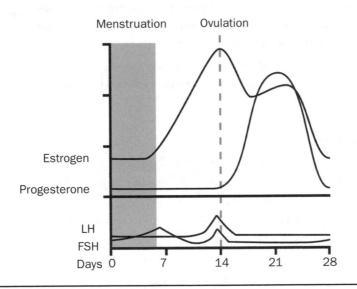

Early in the menstrual cycle, an increased level of a hormone called FSH tells the follicle to ripen and the ovaries to produce estrogen. When estrogen levels peak, the hormone LH is released, triggering ovulation. After ovulation, estrogen and progesterone prepare the lining of the uterus to receive a fertilized egg. If the egg is not fertilized, the hormones drop back to their original levels and menstruation occurs.

Menstruation

Menstruation occurs when the blood vessels supplying the uterine lining undergo spasm or contraction, causing the lining to fall away or be sloughed off. The menstrual blood comes out of the uterus via the cervix and vagina. The fallopian tubes have no role in menstrual bleeding. In general, menstrual blood does not clot. Clotting occurs in the presence of heavy bleeding.

Menstruation usually starts at the age of 11 to 13 and stops at menopause. Menstruation occurs every 28 to 29 days, but any variation between 21 and 37 days is considered normal. Bleeding lasting 7 days or less is considered normal. The heaviest flow is usually in the first 2 to 3 days and the total blood loss is only about 30 mL (2 tablespoons).

Menopause

Menopause is the end of a woman's reproductive life (literally: a **pause** in the **menses**). Medically speaking, you are "menopausal" if you haven't had a period for at least 12 months. The average age of menopause in North America is 51, although it may range from 48 to 52 years.

Natural Menopause

The years leading up to the menopause during which you get "menopausal" symptoms are more correctly called the **perimenopause**. During perimenopause your ovaries gradually shut down and are less and less able to create the normal monthly rise and fall of estrogen. This stimulates higher levels of the brain hormone FSH because there is no estrogen to dampen it down. Periods start to become erratic, with bleeding at odd times of the cycle. Sometimes you will ovulate, sometimes you won't. You may get embarrassing and uncomfortable **hot flashes** (or **flushes**), **night sweats**, or **palpitations** (see More Detail box on page 17). Other symptoms include mood swings, sleep problems, aches and pains, and loss of concentration and mental focus.

After menopause, women are at greater risk for long-term health problems such as osteoporosis and cardiovascular disease because they are no longer protected by estrogen. Low estrogen levels also cause skin to age faster. Sex can be uncomfortable as the vagina is thinner and drier. Weight gain may also become a problem (see page 158).

Whether you view menopause as a normal part of aging or a disease to be cured, it may help to realize that, biologically speaking, menopause is as natural as puberty. The good news is that most women sail through menopause with few problems. Contrary to popular belief, menopause does not cause stress and psychological problems in most healthy women (see page 151) and studies show that some women may, in fact, be more mentally healthy once this milestone has passed. For tips on how to sail through your own menopause, see Chapter 10.

Menopause After Surgery

If you have a hysterectomy but keep your ovaries, you will enter menopause just like a woman with a uterus, except, of course, you will not have to cope with erratic periods—a huge bonus. On the other hand, menopause arrives 1 to 3 years early in some women who have had a hysterectomy, perhaps because of interference with the blood supply to the ovaries. If you experience the classic symptoms of hot flashes, poor sleep, and so on, a simple blood test of your FSH level can confirm that you are in perimenopause. When these symptoms settle down permanently you will know that you have reached menopause.

If you have your ovaries removed during your hysterectomy, and you are not already menopausal, your estrogen levels will drop right away and you will immediately enter menopause. Depending on your age, your physician may recommend **hormone replacement therapy** or **HRT** (see Chapter 12) to reduce your symptoms and the risk of long-term health problems.

Feeling Hot?　　　　　　　　　　　[**MORE DETAIL**]

No one is entirely sure what causes hot flashes or night sweats during the years leading up to menopause. We know that the nervous system is cranking up the body's thermostat and there is a sudden release of "fight or flight" hormones, but it's still uncertain whether this is triggered by low levels of estrogen, high levels of FSH, or something else. Studies have found that physically active women have fewer hot flashes than inactive women, implying that hot flashes may be caused by more than just day-to-day variations in sex hormones.

What Can Go Wrong

Heavy or Abnormal Bleeding

There is no strict medical definition of "abnormal" bleeding, but most women know what is abnormal based on their personal experience. The most bothersome menstrual problem is excessive bleeding (**menorrhagia**) or excessive uterine bleeding occurring at irregular intervals (**metrorrhagia**), or both.

Unusual bleeding should always be checked out because it may be a sign that something needs treatment. **If you are bleeding profusely, consult your doctor immediately or go to the emergency room.** If you lose a lot of blood, you may need intravenous fluid administration or even a blood transfusion. Some profuse bleeding is related to a miscarriage. Even if it is not an emergency, frequent heavy bleeding can lead to **anemia** (see page 39).

If you have the following symptoms, your bleeding is more likely to be abnormal:

- flooding (sudden rush of blood)
- passing blood clots like pieces of liver
- soaking more than 10 sanitary napkins per day
- waking up 2 to 3 times a night to change your pad
- needing overnight sanitary napkins constantly
- bleeding heavily for more than a week
- weakness
- dizziness, tiredness, breathlessness
- fainting or lightheadedness.

Endometrial Hyperplasia

Endometrial hyperplasia occurs because ovulation does not happen. In a normal menstrual cycle, a menstrual period is triggered by the fall in estrogen and progesterone levels about 2 weeks after ovulation (see Figure 1–4). If ovulation fails to occur, the lining of the uterus (endometrium) continues to grow. Over time it becomes thick and fragile and tends to bleed (see Figure 1–5). It can also become cancerous if left untreated. Bleeding related to failure of ovulation is also called **dysfunctional uterine bleeding** or **DUB**. It usually occurs in women under the age of 20 and over the age of 40 and is more common in obese women. DUB is usually treated with **progestin** (a synthetic form of progesterone).

"Tampons? Tampons nothing! It was tampons, pads, bloody underwear—you had to be careful of what you wore. It was really debilitating, really unpleasant."

Anne

Figure 1–5. Endometrial Hyperplasia

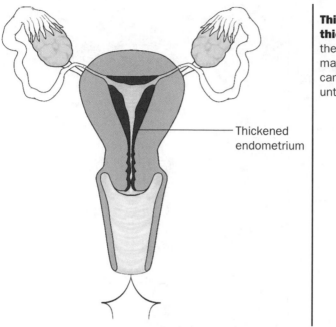

Thickened
endometrium

**This abnormal
thickening** of
the endometrium
may lead to
cancer if left
untreated.

Endometriosis

This painful condition occurs when fragments of the endometrium
migrate out of the uterus and end up elsewhere in the pelvis,
attached to organs such as the ovaries or intestines (see Figure 1–6).
This is possible because the fallopian tubes are open at one end.
The displaced endometrial tissue grows and bleeds in response to
the hormones of the menstrual cycle and causes pain and scarring.

Endometriosis is most common between the ages of 30 and 45,
especially in women who had children late or have never been
pregnant. It is a common cause of infertility. Endometriosis may be

Figure 1–6. Endometriosis

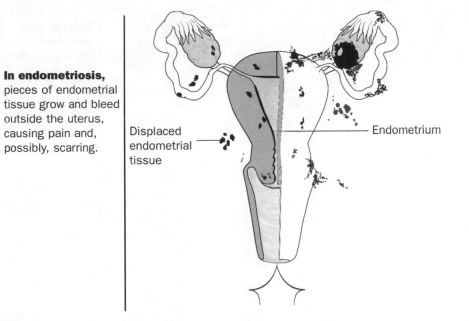

In endometriosis, pieces of endometrial tissue grow and bleed outside the uterus, causing pain and, possibly, scarring.

Displaced endometrial tissue

Endometrium

experienced as pain in the lower abdomen that becomes more severe just before or during a menstrual period. Intercourse, bowel movements, and urination may also be painful.

Endometriosis can be treated with hormones or surgery (see Chapter 3). Hysterectomy is a possibility as a treatment for severe endometriosis if you do not want children or if you have already gone through menopause. Often, both the ovaries and the uterus are removed during the procedure, to be sure of removing all stray endometrial tissue.

Fibroids

Uterine fibroids (myoma or **leiomyoma)** are benign growths of muscle and fibrous tissue at varying depths within the uterine wall (see Figures 1–7 and 1–8). The size of fibroids ranges greatly from that of a pinhead to larger than a football. The largest fibroid ever reported weighed more than 9 kg (20 pounds). Fibroids can make the uterus very large and the woman look pregnant. They do not usually turn into cancer, except in rare cases (a condition called **leiomyosarcoma**).

There are three types of fibroids, depending on their location. **Submucous fibroids** are located inside the uterus, just under the uterine lining. They can cause excessive bleeding, leading to anemia. **Intramural fibroids** are located within the wall of the uterus. **Subserous fibroids** occur under the outer wall of the uterus and bulge outward, giving the uterus a "lumpy, bumpy" appearance.

Fibroids are found in one in four women over age 30 and are twice as common in women of African descent than in Asian or Caucasian women. The cause is unknown, but they appear to grow in response to estrogen and progesterone, so they may increase in size more rapidly in women taking the contraceptive pill or hormone replacement therapy, and they usually stop growing after menopause.

Fibroids are not dangerous in themselves, but they can start to cause annoying, painful, or potentially dangerous problems as they grow larger and press on other organs. Women with small fibroids may be unaware of them, as they produce no or few symptoms. When problems do arise, symptoms include abdominal pain and pain in the buttocks or legs. Large fibroids cause pressure symptoms

"With my fibroids, it was always the same: there was puking, my stomach blew up and I would have to go to the hospital and they would do a vaginal ultrasound. I could be anywhere…once I was at work and they had to rush me to the hospital. You never knew when it was going to flare up. You just took your chances."

Betty

Figure 1–7. Fibroids

Fibroids are benign growths of muscle, like calluses, in the wall of the uterus. They can project outwards (subserous) or into the cavity of the uterus (submucosal). Intramural fibroids are embedded in the wall.

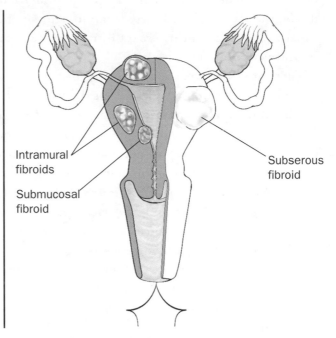

Intramural fibroids

Subserous fibroid

Submucosal fibroid

such as a "bearing down" or a heavy sensation in the pelvic area, frequent urination, and constipation due to pressure against the rectum. Backache is also common. Fibroids can result in infertility or frequent miscarriages. Rapidly growing fibroids, especially fibroids that grow after menopause, need immediate attention.

There are several options for treating fibroids (see Chapters 3 and 7). Small fibroids may not need treatment unless they grow larger. Many women who are close to menopause are able to do nothing, and wait for their fibroids to shrink at menopause. If they are on the inner wall, they can be removed by **hysteroscopy** (page 40). If they are on the outer wall they can be removed by **laparoscopy** (page 42). Other options are **uterine fibroid embolization** (page 108), **myomectomy** (page 116), **myolysis** (page 119) or hysterectomy.

Figure 1–8. Wall of Normal Uterus and Uterus with Fibroids

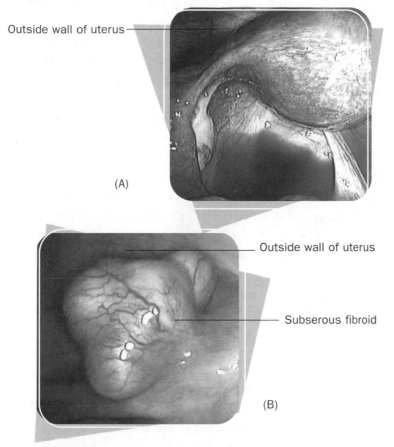

Outside wall of uterus

(A)

Outside wall of uterus

Subserous fibroid

(B)

(A) The wall of a healthy uterus, as seen through a laparoscope.
(B) A fibroid growing out of the wall of the uterus.

Uterine Polyps

Unlike fibroids, which develop from the muscle layers of the
uterus, **uterine polyps** arise from the lining of the uterus, so they
are found on the surface of the cervix or on the inside of the
uterus. Polyps may occur singly or in groups and grow no larger

than about 3 cm (1.25 inches). They are common, especially in pre-menopausal women over age 30, are usually harmless and rarely become cancerous.

The symptoms of uterine polyps are a watery, bloodstained discharge from the vagina and bleeding between periods, after intercourse, or after menopause. Treatment is usually quick and easy. Polyps on the cervix can be removed during a speculum examination (page 32) and uterine polyps can be removed during hysteroscopy (page 40).

Prolapse

Prolapse of the uterus happens when the uterus sags down from its normal location due to weakness and loss of elasticity in its supporting muscles and ligaments due to aging or childbirth (see Figure 1—9). Prolapse is also more likely with conditions that put strain on the pelvic floor and the supporting muscles, such as a chronic cough, obesity, chronic constipation, and heavy lifting. It is more common after menopause.

"My husband would tell me, 'It's not like you're gaining weight, but you know your legs are bigger,' and then I realized they were. When the fibroids were gone I noticed they went back to normal."

Susan

If you have a uterine prolapse, you may be able to feel your cervix low in the vagina and a sensation of pressure or heaviness. Backache and painful intercourse are also common. In severe cases, the cervix may actually protrude out of the vagina. The sagging uterus can pull the rectum or bladder down with it, causing urinary difficulties, infections, or urine leakage with

straining, coughing, or laughing. You may also have difficulty emp-
tying your bowels.

Options for treating mild uterine prolapse include Kegel
exercises (page 168) and estrogen cream applied to the vagina to
strengthen the supporting tissues. Your physician may also suggest a
pessary, a plastic device inserted into the vagina to hold the uterus
in place. Hysterectomy is the choice for a severe prolapse. About 15
percent of all hysterectomies are for uterine prolapse. If you have a
prolapse and still want children, reconstructive surgery may be possible instead of a hysterectomy.

Figure 1–9. Prolapse

(A)

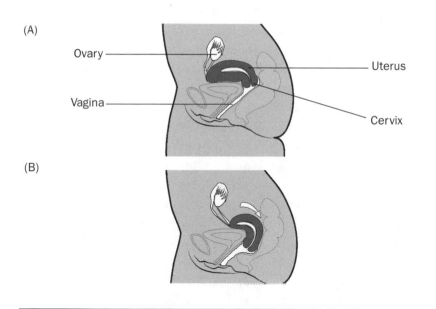

(B)

(A) Uterus in normal position. The uterus is normally held in place by muscles
and ligaments.
(B) Prolapsed uterus. If the muscles and ligaments become weak due to aging
or muscle strain, the uterus may sag downward into the vagina.

Cancer

Cancer of the Cervix

Cancer of the cervix or **cervical cancer** is a common cancer in women, but it is one of the few that can be prevented by regular screening. The screening consists of a simple test called a **cervical smear test** or **Pap test** that is carried out in a doctor's office, in which he or she takes a small sample of cells from the cervix during a normal gynecological checkup. If abnormal cells are found (a condition called **cervical dysplasia**), the abnormal tissue can be removed before it turns cancerous (see page 120). Cervical dysplasia is most common in women age 25 to 35.

Cancer of the cervix is usually found during a routine checkup, as there are few symptoms. Some women may experience abnormal bleeding, especially after intercourse, a watery, bloodstained, offensive-smelling discharge, pain during intercourse, or pelvic pain. If left untreated cervical cancer may spread to the uterus and other organs. Localized cervical cancer is seen most in women age 30 to 40.

Treatment for cervical cancer depends on the severity of the disease. If only a small area is affected and you wish to have children, it may be possible to remove just part of the cervix. More commonly, a hysterectomy will be needed. If you are pre-menopausal, your physician may try to leave your ovaries in, to avoid surgical menopause (page 16). If cervical cancer is found and treated early, nearly all women make a full recovery. If the cancer has spread beyond the cervix, about 3 in 5 women will recover.

Cancer of the Uterus

Cancer of the uterus (**endometrial** or **uterine cancer**) is the most common cancer of the female reproductive organs. It is rare in young women, but is found in approximately 1 in 1,000 women over 50. The cancer arises from the uterine lining (see Figure 1–10). The most

common first sign is bleeding after
menopause, so if this happens to you, see a
physician right away. In the United States,
over 36,000 new cases are discovered each
year. Fortunately, in three-quarters of
them the cancer is still limited to the
uterus, and a hysterectomy will cure the
patient. Compared to Canada and the
United States, endometrial cancer is rarely seen in Asia.

Uterine cancer is more likely in women who are obese or have
never been pregnant. Women with **polycystic ovarian syndrome**
and those who are taking **tamoxifen** for breast cancer treatment or
prevention are also more likely to get endometrial cancer. It is now
well known that taking estrogen without progesterone (**unopposed
estrogen**) is associated with a higher risk of endometrial cancer.

Figure 1–10. Uterine Cancer

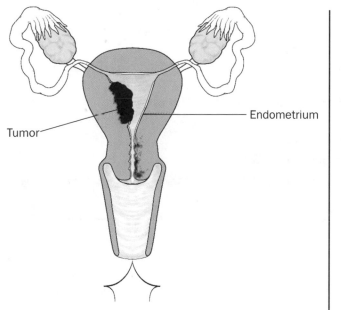

Tumor

Endometrium

**Uterine cancer
starts in the
lining** of the
uterus (the
endometrium)
and can spread
to the ovaries
and other
organs if left
untreated.

For this reason, hormone replacement therapy in women with an intact uterus usually includes progesterone as well as estrogen.

Left untreated, endometrial cancer can spread to the fallopian tubes, ovaries, and other organs. In most women, uterine cancer can be effectively treated with hysterectomy. The ovaries and fallopian tubes are usually removed as well as the uterus. Depending on the severity of the cancer, you may need radiation before or after surgery. Your physician may also recommend chemotherapy if the cancer has spread to lymph nodes.

Bleeding— What Else Might It Be?

[**MORE DETAIL**]

Not all bleeding from the vagina is due to problems with your uterus. Some other common reasons are listed below.

- Miscarriage
- Ectopic pregnancy (pregnancy in the wrong location—outside the womb, usually in a fallopian tube)
- Drugs, e.g., blood thinners heparin and Coumadin, digitalis, and Aspirin
- Herbs, e.g., ginseng, which has estrogen-like activity that can cause bleeding
- Thyroid disorders
- Kidney or liver failure
- Blood-clotting disorders (e.g., **Von Willebrand's disease** or **Factor XI deficiency**)

What Happens Next?

If your physician suspects that you have a problem with your uterus, he or she will carry out tests to find out exactly what is wrong. If your main symptom is excessive bleeding, your first stop will be a blood test to check your blood iron levels, coagulation (blood-clotting) factors, and thyroid hormones. You may also be sent for an ultrasound scan or a hysteroscopy to look inside your uterus, and an endometrial biopsy to take a sample of your uterine lining. All these tests are covered in the next chapter.

Chapter 2

tests and investigations

What Happens in this Chapter

- Your basic pelvic exam
- The facts on anemia
- The inside story on Pap tests, colposcopy, ultrasound, biopsy, D&C, hysteroscopy, and laparoscopy
- What the tests are and what they tell us

There are numerous tests and investigations available to your physician to find out what the problem is. As a first step, he or she will almost certainly carry out a basic pelvic exam and a blood test. You may also be sent for an ultrasound test, to look at your uterus and the ovaries. A Pap test and colposcopy give more detailed information about your cervix, while hysteroscopy and laparoscopy give the full picture on your uterus and other pelvic organs. Once the results of all these investigations are known, you and your physican can decide whether you really need a hysterectomy and, if so, which type.

WHEN YOU FIRST GO AND SEE YOUR PHYSICIAN ABOUT ABNORMAL bleeding or other gynecological symptoms, he or she will first take a complete medical history from you. He or she will be particularly interested in the pattern of your bleeding, as this gives important clues as to the cause. This will usually be followed by a **pelvic examination**. Depending on what is found, your physician will then recommend that you undergo one or more further investigations. This is likely to include a blood test as a first step, followed by an **ultrasound**. Other tests will then follow if your physician feels that they are needed.

The purpose of all these tests is first, to determine whether your bleeding is coming from the uterus, the cervix, the anus, or your bladder, and second, to find out the cause of the bleeding.

It is important to be open and honest and share as much detail as you can with your gynecologist. It may help to write down dates and symptoms before you go. Shed your embarrassment and don't feel intimidated. You are the customer seeking information and appropriate care. Try to be proactive. Ask questions and expect full answers. Most gynecologists these days, both men and women, are sensitive to women's concerns and want to include you in the decision-making, but there are always exceptions. If you don't like the way your doctor responds to your concerns, or you don't trust him or her, change doctors. Remember, it's your body, not the physician's, and your health, not his or hers. You deserve the best care that is out there, and the best quality of life that modern medicine can provide.

"I went through six gynecologists, because every one would say, 'Oh it's nothing, everything is fine.' Meanwhile, I kept having a lot of pain and very irregular periods and a lot of bleeding. One gynecologist just said to me, 'Oh, I always feel weak too;' I was really desperate at that point. The final gynecologist was really concerned and said, 'You really are anemic: I can tell just by looking at you.' He was so concerned he was calling me at home to make sure I was fine."

Silvia

Basic Pelvic Examination

What Is It?

A basic pelvic examination consists of two parts: a **speculum examination** and an **internal examination**. For this, you will be lying on your back with your legs bent (see Figure 2–1). You will need to remove all clothing below the waist. Examination rooms can be cold, though, so if you are wearing socks you may want to keep them on. You can also ask for a blanket.

A speculum consists of two adjustable plastic or metal paddles shaped like a duck's bill that gently stretch the vagina to allow the physician a clear view of the cervix. The physician will gently insert the speculum into your vagina, then gradually open up the "bill." This is not a painful procedure, although the speculum will feel cold unless your physician warms it up first.

Following the speculum examination, your physician will do an internal examination. For this, he or she will insert one or two gloved fingers into your vagina (and sometimes, your rectum) and place the other hand on your lower abdomen. Try to relax if possible: it does not take long and shouldn't be painful. Tense muscles make the examination more difficult for both you and your physician.

Figure 2–1. An Internal Examination

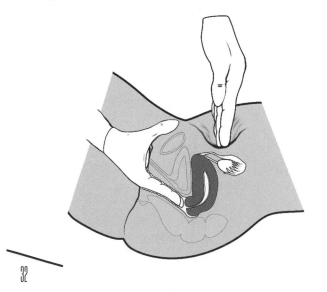

This examination is performed to check the size, shape, and position of the uterus and ovaries.

What Can It Tell Us?

During the speculum examination, your physician will be able to see whether your uterus is sagging (uterine prolapse, see page 24). In order to see how low your uterus will come down, you might be asked to strain or cough.

The internal examination allows the physician to feel the size and shape of your uterus and ovaries, and whether you have other abnormalities in your pelvis. Doctors usually judge the size of the uterus by using pregnancy as a yardstick. For example, a uterus enlarged due to fibroids is called a "12-week-size" uterus if the size is similar to that of a woman who is 12 weeks pregnant. A "20-week-size" uterus reaches the level of the navel. Both internal and external examinations are needed because a uterus smaller than a 12-week size cannot be felt by external abdominal examination alone.

The basic pelvic examination is very useful, but cannot tell the physician everything. For example, only large fibroids can be detected

[S E L F - H E L P]

Help Yourself to Health

Gynecological examinations are hardly a woman's favorite way to spend a morning, but a positive attitude may help—try to think of them as an essential step towards a better life. During an exam, relaxation techniques can be very helpful and give you a sense of control over the situation, despite the somewhat undignified position in which you find yourself. Deep, slow breathing through your nose is a simple and effective way to relax and gives you something to focus on.

this way, and even fibroids as large as 5 cm (2 inches) in diameter are missed three out of four times. If your physician finds that your uterus is slightly bulky, the next step is an ultrasound examination.

Pap Test

What Is It?

During your speculum exam, your physician may do a **Papanicolau** (or Pap) **test**. This involves gently scraping the cervix with a tiny brush or a wooden stick that looks like a long ice cream stick. It should not be painful, and most women don't even feel it. The cells will then be smeared on a glass slide or placed in fluid and sent to the laboratory to be examined under a microscope.

What Can It Tell Us?

This simple test saves millions of lives every year. The laboratory will look for abnormal cells from the cervix, in particular, precancerous cells or cancer cells. If precancerous cells are found (a condition called cervical dysplasia, see page 26) this does not mean you will definitely get cancer. Two out of five cases of cervical dysplasia revert to normal without treatment. However, you will need further tests, including a **colposcopy** (see below), and regular Pap tests every 6 months for the first few years. After that, annual Pap tests are essential.

Normally, you should go to your physician for a Pap test at least once a year, and it is usually part of every well-woman annual checkup.

> **[KEY POINT]**
>
> **If you get a positive Pap test** it does not automatically mean you have cancer of the cervix. More likely, you have a condition called cervical dysplasia, which is simply an early warning that something untoward is starting to happen. It may clear up by itself. If you're unsure what your "positive Pap" means, don't leave your physician's office until you are sure.

Because samples are taken only from the cervix, a Pap test cannot be used to detect cancer in the uterine lining (endometrial cancer) or the ovaries.

Colposcopy

What Is It?

A colposcope is a lighted viewing instrument like a microscope that allows the physician to examine the vagina and cervix more closely. During this test, which lasts about 15 minutes, a speculum will be used to keep the vagina open. The colposcopist will paint various solutions on your cervix to highlight suspicious-looking areas. He or she may also take small tissue samples from the cervix (a **cervical biopsy**). This is usually not too uncomfortable and takes a few more minutes. A biopsy may cause slight spotting or bleeding for a few days.

What Can It Tell Us?

Colposcopy is used to confirm the results of the Pap test. It is not uncommon for a Pap test to give a "false positive"—that is, the Pap test shows an abnormality but nothing is found on colposcopy. Colposcopy will confirm whether you have abnormal cells on your cervix, whether they are cancerous, and how extensive they are.

Colposcopy may also be used during treatment. It gives essential information about the cervix for **laser surgery**, **cryosurgery**, and **loop electrosurgical excision** (**LEEP**). Chapter 7 describes these procedures.

Ultrasound Test

What Is It?

Ultrasound examination is a simple test using sound waves to bounce an image back to a television screen. Ultrasound reveals the organs in "slices" so the images are hard to interpret unless you know what you're looking for. With ultrasound, the body is not exposed to radiation. There are several types of ultrasound examination.

During **abdominal ultrasound**, the technician will rub a sound transmitter gently over your abdomen to display your internal organs from "the top." Abdominal ultrasound is uncomfortable because you

Help Yourself to... Another Glass of Water

You'll be told to drink up to seven glasses of water before you come for your ultrasound, but one very large glass (at least 500 mL or 16oz) about an hour before is usually enough. Although it's uncomfortable, hang in there. If your bladder is not full when you arrive at the clinic, your ultrasound may be canceled and you will have to return another day. The technician will work fast and you'll be allowed to go the bathroom immediately after your abdominal ultrasound is over.

need a very full bladder for this procedure (see Self-Help box). The lubricating gel may also feel a little cold. A full bladder pushes the intestines out of the way, allowing the technician to see your uterus properly.

Vaginal ultrasound gives more precise images of your reproductive organs from "the inside." Because vaginal ultrasound is closer to your internal organs, the images are clearer and the doctor will be able to make a more accurate diagnosis. For this test, a specially designed sound transmitter is placed inside your vagina. It is first covered with a condom to reduce the risk of disease transmission. Your bladder does not need to be full, so you will be allowed to go the bathroom first. Your hips are slightly raised for this test, so it can be a little uncomfortable, especially if you have back problems.

Saline instillation ultrasound or **sonohysterography** allows easier detection of any growths inside the uterus. Because the cavity of the womb is usually collapsed, fibroids or polyps may be squashed flat and not clearly visible on ultrasound. In this technique, a sterile solution is introduced into the uterus, distending it and allowing the surface details to be seen. The downside is that the uterus doesn't like to be stretched, and may respond by cramping down. Painkillers such as ibuprofen or ASA (e.g., Aspirin) taken beforehand can help with this. There is also a slight risk of infection, so tell your physician beforehand if you have had a pelvic infection, in which case you may be advised against the test or prescribed antibiotics as a precaution.

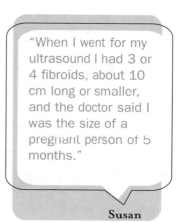

"When I went for my ultrasound I had 3 or 4 fibroids, about 10 cm long or smaller, and the doctor said I was the size of a pregnant person of 5 months."

Susan

What Can It Tell Us?

Ultrasound will give a clear picture of your uterus and ovaries and tell you whether there is anything suspicious. The doctor will be able to measure the thickness of the uterine lining, or the size of a fibroid, to the nearest millimeter. However, ultrasound cannot definitely tell whether the lining is normal, pre-cancerous or cancerous. An **endometrial biopsy** is needed for this. If an endometrial biopsy is not possible, **a dilation and curettage (D&C)** may be performed instead. If your physician suspects fibroids and the ultrasound did not give him or her enough information, the next step may be a hysteroscopy, which reveals fibroids on the inside of the uterus, or a laparoscopy, which shows fibroids on the outside of the uterus. All these procedures are described below.

Endometrial Biopsy

What Is It?

If your vaginal ultrasound shows that your uterine lining is thick, your doctor will advise an endometrial biopsy. This simple, in-office procedure takes less than a minute. A thin plastic tube like a fine drinking straw is inserted into your uterus through the cervix, and gentle suction is used to remove a sample of the uterine lining. You will experience a few minutes of cramping afterward. The tissue is then sent to the laboratory for staining and examination under a microscope.

What Can It Tell Us?

An endometrial biopsy is simple, but it's packed with information. It will show whether the uterine lining is normal, or very thick (endometrial hyperplasia), or contains cancer or precancerous cells.

Dilation and Curettage (D&C)

What Is It?

A D&C is a short surgical procedure that involves removing the inner lining of the uterus with a spoon-shaped scraper called a **curette**. A suction device may be used as an alternative. The tissue that is removed is sent to the laboratory for analysis. A D&C may be done in your physician's office under local anesthesia, or in a hospital or ambulatory surgery center under general or regional anesthesia.

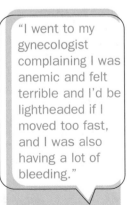

"I went to my gynecologist complaining I was anemic and felt terrible and I'd be lightheaded if I moved too fast, and I was also having a lot of bleeding."

Anne

Before your D&C, the physician will perform a pelvic examination. He or she will then gradually open (dilate) the cervix using smooth rods of increasing sizes. Once the cervix is about 1 cm (1/2 inch) dilated, the curettage will be performed. Most D&Cs take about 15 minutes and you will go home the same day. You may have cramping for a day or so and spotting for several weeks. If you bleed heavily for more than a week afterward, see your physician.

Anemia—The Inside Story

[**MORE DETAIL**]

Oxygen is carried throughout your body in red blood cells, attached to an iron-containing pigment called **hemoglobin**. If you experience vaginal bleeding for a long time or have excessively heavy bleeding, you may have a deficiency of red blood cells or hemoglobin. This is called anemia. Because hemoglobin delivers oxygen to your tissues, if you are anemic you may feel very tired, weak and dizzy, breathless, and faint.

The normal hemoglobin level is 120 to 160 g/L (grams per liter of blood) and the blood-iron level (**ferritin**) is 46 to 230 µg/L (micrograms per liter). In women with uterine bleeding, the hemoglobin level can be normal, but the ferritin level very low—sometimes lower than 10 µg/L—so measurement of ferritin is important.

If you are very anemic, it is better to postpone your surgery until your levels are normal. Treatment of anemia before surgery can include iron pills, medicine to stop your periods, or, occasionally, injection of a hormone called **erythropoietin** that stimulates red blood cell production. For more on anemia before surgery, see page 70.

Dilation and curettage is an all-purpose gynecological technique. As well as being a diagnostic test, for many years it was the standard treatment for heavy uterine bleeding. It is also used to prevent hemorrhage after a miscarriage by removing traces of the placenta, and to terminate a pregnancy.

What Can It Tell Us?

Sometimes, an endometrial biopsy cannot be performed because the cervix is too narrow, therefore it is necessary to dilate the cervix. A

D&C can detect many problems in the uterus, including fibroids, uterine cancer, and cervical polyps. If a simple problem is found, such as polyps, it can also treat them at the same time. The disadvantage of a D&C is that it is a "blind technique," which means the doctor does not see what is being scraped. Studies have shown that about a quarter of the uterine lining can be missed by a D&C. For this reason, endometrial sampling or hysteroscopy are increasingly used in place of a D&C.

Hysteroscopy

What Is It?

A hysteroscope is a small, fiber-optic telescope attached to a camera that is used to see inside the uterus. It is inserted through the vagina and the cervix and no incision is needed (see Figure 2–2). Gas or a clear fluid is used to expand the uterus for a better view and the pictures show up on a TV screen. Hysteroscopy takes about 15 minutes and can be done in your doctor's office, if he or she is set up for it. It can be done under local, spinal, or general anesthesia.

[**KEY POINT**]

If your doctor recommends a D&C for diagnosis, ask for an endometrial biopsy first, or, better yet, hysteroscopy. These techniques are less invasive and give more information than a D&C.

A good approach is to combine hysteroscopy with a **fractional D&C**. In this procedure, your physician will scrape first the cervix and then the uterine lining and send the scrapings to the laboratory in two separate jars. This will pinpoint the exact location of any abnormality.

As well as being a diagnostic technique, hysteroscopy is also used for treatment (see Chapter 7).

What Can It Tell Us?

Hysteroscopy gives your gynecologist a clear view of the inside of the uterus and allows him or her to see any fibroids, polyps, or suspicious tissue. If endometrial cancer is found, the separate scrapings from a fractional D&C will tell you if the cancer is limited to the uterus or has spread to the cervix.

Hysteroscopy cannot show the outside of the uterus. For this, a laparoscopy is needed (see page 42).

Figure 2–2. Hysteroscopy

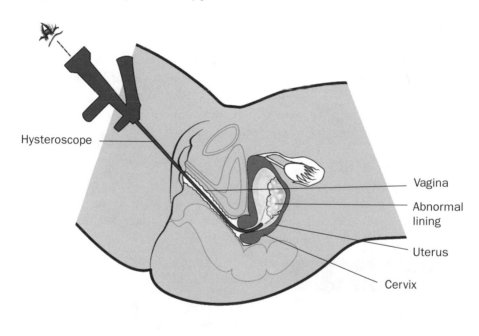

A small telescope is inserted into the uterus for this procedure, which allows the physician to check the inside of the uterus for fibroids, polyps, or other abnormalities.

Laparoscopy

What Is It?

In this technique, a long telescope with a light on the end (called a **laparoscope**) is inserted into your abdomen to examine your uterus and other pelvic organs (see Figure 6–3 on page 88). Laparoscopy involves a small incision, so it is considered a minor surgical procedure. It is almost always carried out under a general anesthetic so it will need to be done in a hospital or surgical center.

As well as being used for diagnosis, laparoscopy can be used as a "minimally invasive" technique for many surgeries, including hysterectomy. As it involves only small incisions, recovery is often much faster. For more on laparoscopic hysterectomy, see page 86.

> "My doctor did an ultrasound and it seemed like endometriosis, so he said let's keep an eye on it. [A few months later] I wasn't getting on well, so they did a diagnostic laparoscopy and excision of the endometriotic implants."
>
> Silvia

What Can It Tell Us?

Laparoscopy gives a clear view of the outside of the uterus so it can be used to diagnose fibroids that project outward from the uterus instead lying inside. It is also the only way to accurately diagnose endometriosis and take a look at the tubes or ovaries.

Blood Test

What Is It?

A blood test is routine if you go to see your physician about abnormal uterine bleeding. Most women are familiar with this procedure, in which a blood technician uses a needle to take a small sample of blood from a vein in the arm. The blood then goes to the laboratory for analysis.

What Can It Tell Us?

Your small blood sample is packed with information. The laboratory will look for hemoglobin, red cell, and ferritin levels to see if you are anemic (see More Detail box on page 39). The test will also check whether your blood can clot normally. Problems with blood clotting can cause uterine bleeding—and uncontrollable bleeding after surgery. The lab will measure levels of small cell fragments called **platelets**, which are key elements in blood clotting, and levels of coagulation factors, the proteins in your blood that make blood clot. Although problems with blood clotting such as Von Willebrand's disease or Factor XI deficiency are rare, they can go undetected for many years.

An underactive thyroid gland, a condition called **hypothyroidism**, can cause excessive uterine bleeding. The most sensitive blood test to diagnose hypothyrodism is **TSH** or **thyroid stimulating hormone** measurement. TSH is a hormone from the pituitary gland that is elevated in hypothyroidism to stimulate your "lazy" thyroid gland.

What Happens Next?

In most women, a combination of these tests will give a clear picture of what is wrong. The next step is deciding on the best treatment. Unless you have uterine cancer, there are many options available to you in addition to hysterectomy, so take the time to discuss them with your physician and don't be rushed into anything. Chapter 7 gives detailed information on the alternatives and Chapter 3 gives you some help deciding between them and hysterectomy.

If your diagnosis is still unclear, or you feel uncertain about it, or you simply do not feel comfortable with your gynecologist's recommendations for treatment, do not be afraid to seek a second, third, fourth, or even fifth opinion. One of the author's patients had seen seven other gynecologists before coming to him for an opinion.

If you decide on a hysterectomy, you may request referral to another gynecologic surgeon who is expert in the type of hysterectomy that you want. The different types of hysterectomy are discussed in the next chapter. If you need a radical hysterectomy for uterine cancer, you should be referred to a gynecologic oncologist—a gynecologist who is trained to do surgery for cancer of the reproductive organs.

Chapter 3

is hysterectomy right for you?

What Happens in this Chapter

- How to make your decision
- A brief overview of the different types of hysterectomy
- Pros and cons of the alternatives
- The upsides and downsides of hysterectomy
- Hysterectomy myths

Unless you have invasive cancer or very severe bleeding, hysterectomy should no longer be seen as the answer to every gynecological problem. Heavy periods, fibroids, polyps, mild prolapse, endometriosis, and many other gynecological conditions can be helped by other procedures and drugs. Deciding between them all can be difficult, especially if your physician is convinced that hysterectomy is the best route and you're not. This chapter aims to help you sort through the confusion and reach a decision that is right for you.

The Hysterectomy Decision

HYSTERECTOMY IS THE SECOND MOST COMMON PROCEDURE performed on women in North America—second only to cesarean sections—and around 1 in 4 women will reach the age of 60 without her uterus. Many people have questioned whether all these hysterectomies are really necessary. Studies in the 1990s showed that up to 2 in 3 women underwent the procedure without good medical reasons. Clearly, hysterectomy means big business—and big controversy.

If you are told you need a hysterectomy, it's important to keep a clear head. Ask lots of questions (some suggestions are on page 73). Explore your options. Talk to other women, go on the Internet, get a second opinion—or a third, or fourth. Do not agree to a hysterectomy until you fully understand why you are having it, why the alternatives may not work for you, and what you can expect from the procedure.

Once your ultrasound and other tests have confirmed that you might need a hysterectomy, your physician will make a recommendation based on her or his experience with patients whose medical condition is similar to yours, the number of factors in your life that may affect your condition, his or her familiarity with a certain technique, and his or her knowledge of the most recent scientific studies.

> "I have a great belief in instinct. You know. You know if you need this. And you shouldn't be talked into it by a physician."
>
> **Anne**

> "I shouldn't have to go on the Internet and do my homework. If there are negative sides to the alternatives, well, my doctor could have told me about that, but he didn't. Nothing. I wasn't given a choice. And that's sad, because this is his specialty. When I told him, 'Listen, I'm not sure if I want to do a hysterectomy because of all the stories I heard,' he said, 'That's all in people's heads.'"
>
> **Susan**

Hysterectomy may be a medical necessity, for example if you have endometrial cancer or life-threatening bleeding. If not, the decision is less clear-cut and your physician should discuss alternate treatments with you before the decision is made to proceed with the hysterectomy. If you do decide on hysterectomy, again, there are several alternative ways to perform it. If there is no particular medical reason to choose one treatment over another, the decision may depend on practical considerations, such as locally available hospital resources, the comfort of your surgeon with a certain surgical procedure, and how quickly you need to return to work.

Chapter 6 covers the different types of hysterectomy and Chapter 7 summarizes the advantages and disadvantages of the alternatives—drug treatment, endometrial ablation, uterine fibroid embolization, and myomectomy. This chapter tries to pull it all together to help you make an informed decision about your treatment.

How to Decide? [**MORE DETAIL**]

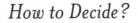

- In general, it's best to start with the least invasive treatment and go on to more invasive procedures if necessary.
- Your own health condition may mean that one or more of the alternatives is not available to you.
- If in doubt, get a second (or third) opinion from another physician. Tell them you are seeking another opinion. This is normal. Your family doctor or friends will be able to suggest alternate physicians.
- As with all illnesses, your condition can change over time and you may need to revise your decision.
- You are entitled to change your mind beforehand if you feel that you have made a wrong choice.
- Remember, you cannot undo surgery!

What Can You Do?

Most conditions have several possible treatments and your options will depend on your own personal circumstances. Start here with your condition. Once you know what treatments are available to you, check out page 48 for a summary of the pros and cons of each.

What have you got?	What are your options?
Menstrual Problems/Heavy Bleeding/Endometrial Hyperplasia	• Wait and see • Drug treatments • Progesterone intrauterine system • Endometrial ablation • Hysterectomy
Uterine Fibroids	• Wait and see • Fibroid embolization • Myomectomy • Hysterectomy (abdominal, vaginal or laparoscopic, subtotal or total)
Benign Uterine Polyps	• Do nothing if no symptoms • Removal during hysteroscopy
Endometriosis	• Drug treatments • Hysterectomy (abdominal, vaginal or laparoscopic) with or without removal of the ovaries • Laparoscopic exision
Prolapsed Uterus	• Kegel exercises (if very mild) • Estrogen therapy • Pessary • Total hysterectomy (especially vaginal) • Reconstructive surgery
Pelvic Inflammatory Disease	• Antibiotics • Total hysterectomy (rarely)
Isolated Cervical Cancer (not spread)	• Total hysterectomy
Cervical Cancer (spread)	• Total/radical hysterectomy (+ ovary removal unless pre-menopausal)
Uterine Cancer	• Total/radical hysterectomy + ovary removal
High Risk of Uterine or Ovarian Cancer	• Total hysterectomy + ovary removal

Your Options—Pros and Cons

This table summarizes the advantages and disadvantages of each treatment. The pros and cons of the alternatives to hysterectomy are discussed more fully in Chapter 7.

Treatment	Advantages	Disadvantages
Wait and See (page 101)	• No surgery • Buys time for self-help measures or drugs	• Symptoms may continue
Non-hormone Drugs (page 104)	• Easy to take • Effective for many women	• Side effects • May not be enough
Hormone Treatments (page 105)	• Estrogen/proges-terone easy to take • Effective for many women	• Side effects • Risk of blood clots • Can't be used in smokers over 35
Progesterone Intrauterine System (page 105)	• Convenient • Reduces bleeding in many women	• Bleeding may be irregular • Side effects • Risk of pelvic infection, ectopic pregnancy, ovarian cysts • Cost
Pessary (page 121)	• Non-surgical • Simple • Reversible	• Temporary measure • Discomfort, chafing, inconvenience
Endometrial Ablation (page 112)	• No hospital stay • No incisions • For 1 in 5, no bleeding • For 3 in 5, bleeding is reduced • Rapid recovery	• Risk, discomfort, inconvenience • 1 in 5 show no improvement • Hysterectomy still needed in 20 to 30 percent of patients within 3 years • Pregnancy no longer advisable
Fibroid Embolization (page 109)	• Non-surgical option • Very effective for heavy bleeding • Shrinks fibroids permanently	• Risk, discomfort, inconvenience • Triggers early menopause in 1 in 100 women • Decreases fertility • More fibroids may grow

Treatment	Advantages	Disadvantages
Myomectomy (page 116)	• Pregnancy still possible although cesarean may be needed	• Major surgery • Risk, discomfort, inconvenience • Technically difficult • High blood loss • More fibroids may grow • Repeat surgery is needed in 15 percent of women
Vaginal Hysterectomy (page 89)	• Ideal for uterine prolapse • No visible scar • Shorter hospital stay and more comfortable recovery compared to abdominal hysterectomy	• Technically difficult for large fibroids • Doctor can't look around the pelvis easily • Difficult to remove ovaries • Cervix is removed
Laparoscopic Hysterectomy (page 86)	• Shorter hospital stay and recovery compared to abdominal hysterectomy	• Not suitable for cancer or large fibroids
Abdominal Hysterectomy (page 86)	• Necessary for large fibroids	• Large scar • Longest hospital stay and recovery
Subtotal Hysterectomy (page 50)	• Cervix is retained • Less chance of infection	• Not suitable for cervical cancer • Cannot be done by vaginal route • Some women continue to have monthly "period"
Total/Radical Hysterectomy (pages 51 and 52)	• Necessary for cancer of the uterus or cervix	• Cervix is removed
Total/Radical Hysterectomy + Ovary Removal (pages 51 and 52)	• Reduces risk of ovarian cancer • Necessary for ovarian cancer or severe endometriosis	• Cervix is removed • Menopause begins right away (surgical menopause)

What Is a Hysterectomy?

Hysterectomy involves surgically removing the uterus and there are several different types of hysterectomy procedures (see also Figure 6–1 on page 85).

Subtotal or Partial Hysterectomy

This procedure leaves the cervix in place.

A subtotal hysterectomy is an option if you have fibroids or heavy uterine bleeding. It is not suitable for women with cancer of the cervix or uterus, for obvious reasons. It's also not an option for uterine prolapse.

The advantage of subtotal hysterectomy compared to total hysterectomy is that it does not disturb the anatomy of the pelvic floor. In theory, this might prevent sagging of the vagina (prolapse) or the bladder in the future. There is also less risk of injury to the urinary tract and reduced chance of infection after the procedure, as bacteria from the vagina are less likely to contaminate the area of the

How Long Are You Staying?　　　　[MORE DETAIL]

Type of Hysterectomy	Time in Hospital	Time to Return to Work
Laparoscopic	0 to 2 days	2 to 4 weeks
Vaginal	0 to 2 days	2 to 4 weeks
Abdominal	3 to 5 days	4 to 8 weeks

surgery. Some women prefer to have their cervix left in the belief that sexual function is less likely to be affected. Evidence shows, however, that most women have improved sexual function after hysterectomy, whether or not their cervix is removed (see pages 146-150).

The disadvantage of subtotal hysterectomy compared to total hysterectomy is the theoretical risk of cervical cancer in the future, although with regular Pap screening this has now fallen to one-third its old rate—to only 3 in 1,000. In addition, some women may require additional surgery due to prolapse of the cervix or bleeding.

Total Hysterectomy

This involves removal of the entire uterus, including the cervix. If the ovaries are left in place, you will continue to ovulate, but, of course, you will not experience a menstrual period. If your ovaries are removed as well, this is called a **total hysterectomy with salpingo-oophorectomy**.

A total hysterectomy is needed for a uterine prolapse and for cervical or uterine cancer.

The advantages and disadvantages of a total hysterectomy compared to the alternative therapies are covered on pages 55-60.

Should You Keep Your Ovaries?

In women with uterine fibroids or abnormal uterine bleeding, routine removal of normal ovaries is no longer recommended—unless you are approaching 50 years old. Women with ovarian cancer or endometriosis will almost certainly have their ovaries removed. You may have heard that in up to 1 in 2 women the ovaries stop working after hysterectomy anyway, so you

"I decided to do my hysterectomy mostly to get my ovaries out and decrease my risk of ovarian cancer. By the age of 55 I'd already had two primary cancers, so I felt like a sitting duck."

Dawn

may as well have them removed. In fact, recent studies dispute these findings, so the decision really hinges on your risk of ovarian cancer.

The downside of removing your ovaries before your own natural menopause is that you suddenly enter **surgical menopause** and menopausal hot flushes and night sweats will start. Your risk of heart disease and osteoporosis also starts to climb. Because the average age of menopause is around 50, women who have their ovaries removed at the age of 40 may lose 10 years of normal ovarian function. After menopause, however, the ovaries do not produce substantial amounts of hormone and removal of the ovaries may be reasonable.

The advantage of having your ovaries removed is that you no longer run the risk of ovarian cancer, so if you have a strong family history of ovarian cancer or a personal history of breast, colon, or rectal cancer, removal of the ovaries is worth considering. However, the risk of developing ovarian cancer if you choose to keep your ovaries is fairly small—about 1 in 140.

Radical Hysterectomy

A radical hysterectomy involves removing all surrounding tissues including the top of the vagina, as well as the uterus, and is generally reserved for cancer of the cervix. The tubes and ovaries may be spared in younger women.

Surgical Routes

As is described in more detail in Chapter 6, there are three possible routes for your hysterectomy: through your abdomen in the usual way, through your vagina, or via laparoscopy (keyhole surgery).

Abdominal Hysterectomy

The abdominal route is needed for cancer or if the fibroids are very large.

Vaginal Hysterectomy

Vaginal hysterectomy involves removing the uterus through the vagina (see Figure 6-4 on page 90) and is the obvious choice for women with prolapse of the uterus. However, it is also an option for other conditions in certain kinds of patients. If you don't have cancer, and your uterus is easily accessible and "mobile" (not too firmly attached to other organs), vaginal hysterectomy may be worth considering. The advantage is that you will avoid any incisions in your abdomen. However, bear in mind that vaginal hysterectomy is not an option if you want to keep your cervix.

Laparoscopic Hysterectomy

Laparoscopy may be a good route if:
- you have a non-cancerous uterus of less than 16-weeks size
- you have persistant pelvic pain
- you have endometriosis
- your surgeon is comfortable with laparoscopic hysterectomy

Making Your Decision on Surgical Routes

Compared to abdominal hysterectomy, vaginal hysterectomy and hysterectomy by laparoscopy are associated with shorter hospital stays and faster recoveries. However, not all women are candidates for these minimally invasive approaches. Whether they are right for you depends on the reason for hysterectomy and also on the expertise of the surgeon with the procedure.

Your doctor will weigh the risks and benefits of each surgical approach and discuss it with you.

Are the Alternatives Right for Me?

The alternative procedures to hysterectomy are shown on pages 48–49. Uterine fibroid embolization involves shrinking the fibroids by blocking their blood supply with tiny beads. **Endometrial ablation** is a procedure that destroys the lining of the uterus. Myomectomy is a surgery that destroys fibroids while leaving the uterus intact. (For a detailed discussion of these procedures, see Chapter 7.)

Uterine fibroid embolization may be a better option for you than hysterectomy, myomectomy, or endometrial ablation, if you have uterine fibroids that are bothering you, you do not wish to undergo hysterectomy, and have no desire for more children. It is not recommended for cancer.

> "That was my goal with embolization— to do something that would get me to menopause when my fibroids would shrink anyway. I figured if I could do something that would take me there, then I wouldn't have to worry."
>
> Susan

Endometrial ablation may be the better choice if you simply have heavy bleeding with no obvious cause (such as fibroids) and do not want a hysterectomy or children. You will need to understand that the results might be temporary.

Myomectomy is the treatment of choice if you have large or numerous fibroids and still want to have children. If you have more than three fibroids larger than 5 cm (2 inches) buried in the wall of the uterus, you will need an abdominal myomectomy. If you have no more than three, you may be able to have laparoscopic myomectomy. Hysteroscopic myomectomy (via the vagina) may be done for relatively small fibroids in the uterine cavity.

A Lifesaver

If you suffer from cancer of the uterus, cervix, or ovaries, hysterectomy is necessary. By removing the cancer, hysterectomy may completely cure you, depending on how advanced your disease is.

Hysterectomy also saves lives in cases of severe, uncontrolled bleeding, for instance, as a result of childbirth or a blood-clotting disorder, or if the uterus is severely infected.

Long-Lasting Results

Hysterectomy immediately stops uterine bleeding and the results are permanent. By contrast, following endometrial ablation, about 1 woman in 4 eventually goes on to need a hysterectomy.

Best Option for Uterine Prolapse

Severe uterine prolapse is best treated with hysterectomy via the vagina although reconstructive surgery may also be possible to preserve the uterus. Other alternatives are not as effective, although they may work as an interim measure. The best of these is a vaginal pessary, a doughnut-shaped device that is inserted into the vagina to support the sagging uterus. However, it is often impractical and inconvenient. It has to be removed every night, washed, and reinserted the next morning. The vagina can get sore and infected and occasionally the pessary gets stuck (or forgotten). Vaginal hysterectomy, along with surgical repair of the sagging organs, corrects the problem.

Quality of Life Improvements

Hysterectomy can improve quality of life by eliminating pain and bleeding. A recent study at the University of Maryland involving

> "With the constant, constant bleeding I felt like I had no control over anything—I felt completely useless. I told my gynecologist, we have to think about me—I'm not well. What are the chances for me to meet anyone and have a baby? If it's not meant to be, it won't happen. He felt bad about it, because he said to me, 'Well, I'm really, really sorry,' and I said, 'Don't worry, it's not easy but there's no choice at this point.' And he looked at me and said, 'No, and we have to do something fast because your situation is really precarious right now.'"
>
> **Silvia**

almost 1,300 women tracked the women's experiences of hysterectomy beforehand and 3, 6, 12, 18, and 24 months after their surgery. The results were published in the *American Journal of Obstetrics and Gynecology* in 2000. The study found that after 2 years, 94 percent of the women said the results were better than or as expected, and 82 percent said their health had improved since their hysterectomy.

Hysterectomy is a better option for you than myomectomy, uterine fibroid embolization, or endometrial ablation if you have:

[**MORE DETAIL**]

- cancer of the uterus, cervix, fallopian tube, or ovary (radical or abdominal hysterectomy)
- uterine prolapse (vaginal hysterectomy)
- a massively enlarged uterus due to uterine fibroids and you do not want any more children (abdominal hysterectomy).

The Downsides of Hysterectomy

Invasive Procedure

Like other surgical procedures, hysterectomy is an invasive procedure, which means it requires an incision, is fairly hard on your body, and recovery takes several weeks. Hysterectomy varies from the minimally invasive vaginal and laparoscopy techniques to a more invasive abdominal hysterectomy. The results, however, are permanent. By contrast, you might undergo a myomectomy procedure, which has a similar recovery time, only to have your fibroids grow back.

General Anesthesia

Uterine fibroid embolization requires only sedation, and endometrial ablation can be done under general, regional or local anesthesia. By contrast, laparoscopic, abdominal hysterectomy and abdominal myomectomy almost always require general anesthesia. Vaginal hysterectomy may be performed under general or regional anesthesia.

More Chance of a Blood Transfusion

A blood transfusion is rarely needed for hysterectomy (about 1 to 2 percent of non-cancer procedures), but it is more common than in alternative techniques, with the exception of abdominal myomectomy. Myomectomy can involve quite high blood loss, so if you're considering it, also consider one or more blood conservation options that can be planned in advance such as blood banking (see page 70).

Longer Hospital Stay

The hospital stay depends on the type of hysterectomy procedure, but it will be longer than for an alternative approach—again, with the exception of myomectomy. For example, you will usually be in hospital no longer than 2 days following a laparoscopic hysterectomy, or a vaginal hysterectomy, and 3 to 5 days following an abdominal hysterectomy or abdominal myomectomy. Alternative procedures such as endometrial ablation do not require hospitalization. Although women often go home the same day after uterine artery embolization, if severe pain is experienced they will be kept overnight to ensure that pain is under control.

Longer Recovery

You may take longer recovering from hysterectomy than from one of the alternatives, especially if you had an abdominal hysterectomy, in which case the recovery time is several weeks. Recovery time is shorter after vaginal and laparoscopic hysterectomy (you may be back to work in 2 to 3 weeks) but it is still likely to be longer than after endometrial ablation or uterine fibroid embolization.

It May Not Work

Hysterectomy is very effective for cancer, and is a permanent, effective solution for fibroids, prolapse, and heavy bleeding. However, for a number of other gynecological problems—such as long-term pelvic pain and endometriosis—there is a risk that you may undergo the procedure without curing your symptoms. The University of Maryland study showed that, although 9 out of 10 women reported that they were "totally recovered" 2 years after hysterectomy, 1 in 10 women had no change in their symptoms.

Other Risks

The risk of having major complications—unwanted medical events— after hysterectomy is greater than after an alternative procedure (see More Detail box, page 60).

Earlier Menopause

Even if the ovaries are not removed, some studies show that as many as 1 in 2 women still stop producing hormones after a hysterectomy, presumably due to disruption of the blood supply. This may depend on the kind of hysterectomy procedure because other studies show that hysterectomy has no effect on the ovaries. However, it is a risk worth considering.

Bladder and Bowel Problems

There is a slight risk that the nerves to your bladder will be cut and urinary sensations lost. Urinary incontinence is also a possibility, due to damage to the pelvic floor. The bowels become obstructed with scar tissue in up to 4 in 1000 women who have had a hysterectomy (see page 176).

Infection

As with all surgeries, an infection is a possibility after hysterectomy. However, the use of preventive antibiotics has reduced the rate of serious infections to less than 1 percent for all types of hysterectomy.

Sexual Difficulties

Major sexual problems after hysterectomy are rare and not the experience of most women, as shown by a recent well-run study that demonstrated sex actually improved overall after the procedure (see page 148). However, you may be one of the unlucky ones. Sex could potentially be affected by nerve damage, scar tissue in the vagina making intercourse painful (especially if you had vaginal repairs in addition to total hysterectomy), vaginal dryness due to surgical menopause, or emotional factors.

"I wouldn't recommend this to a 30-year-old, but at my age, with my bleeding issues, forget it. Why would I want that? Yuck! I can't imagine how anyone can consider it 'feminine' to have to stuff your purse full of pads, tampons and be very careful what you wear. I could tell you stories—sitting in a restaurant I could barely get up, waiting for everyone to leave just in case. It was awful. This is not feminine. This is torture."

Anne

Emotional Difficulties

Emotional problems are common after any major procedure and especially after hysterectomy, when some women mourn the loss of what they view as their "femininity." However, as discussed on pages 150–151, this is a passing phase in the experience of most women, many of whom are relieved to find their lives are now free of pain and inconvenience.

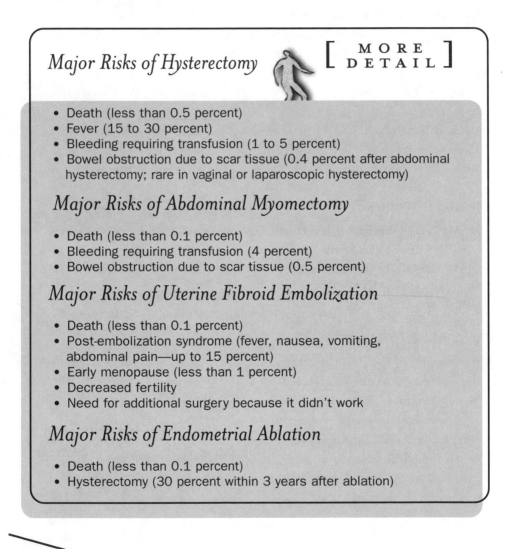

Major Risks of Hysterectomy [MORE DETAIL]

- Death (less than 0.5 percent)
- Fever (15 to 30 percent)
- Bleeding requiring transfusion (1 to 5 percent)
- Bowel obstruction due to scar tissue (0.4 percent after abdominal hysterectomy; rare in vaginal or laparoscopic hysterectomy)

Major Risks of Abdominal Myomectomy

- Death (less than 0.1 percent)
- Bleeding requiring transfusion (4 percent)
- Bowel obstruction due to scar tissue (0.5 percent)

Major Risks of Uterine Fibroid Embolization

- Death (less than 0.1 percent)
- Post-embolization syndrome (fever, nausea, vomiting, abdominal pain—up to 15 percent)
- Early menopause (less than 1 percent)
- Decreased fertility
- Need for additional surgery because it didn't work

Major Risks of Endometrial Ablation

- Death (less than 0.1 percent)
- Hysterectomy (30 percent within 3 years after ablation)

Hysterectomy Myths

When deciding whether to have a hysterectomy, it is worth remembering that more myths surround this procedure than any other. Here are a few of them:

- **If you doctor says you need it, then you need it.** *In fact:* Nine out of 10 hysterectomies are "elective," i.e., done to improve quality of life, but are not essential.

- **Gynecologists ignore women's preferences.** *In fact:* There are exceptions, but most gynecologists, both men and women, will go with a woman's own preference if medically possible.

- **Hysterectomy doesn't work.** *In fact:* Only about 8 percent of women are still experiencing the same symptoms after 2 years; in the vast majority (96 percent) the procedure mostly or completely resolves their symptoms.

- **Male physicians are more likely to recommend hysterectomy.** *In fact:* When age is taken out of the equation, male and female physicians recommend hysterectomy at an equal rate.

- **Alternative procedures offer a faster recovery.** Well, yes and no. A trouble-free vaginal or laparoscopic hysterectomy might have a much faster recovery than an endometrial abla- tion that gets complicated. It all depends on how well the procedure goes.

- **Hysterectomy ruins your sex life.** *In fact:* Although some women are unfortunate, a recent study showed that hysterec- tomy actually *improved sex* overall, presumably by removing bleeding, bloating, pain, and other "unsexy" symptoms.

- **Hysterectomy causes depression.** *In fact:* There is no evidence that hysterectomy for good medical reasons causes emotional problems in women with no prior emotional difficulties. Women who suffer afterward tend to be those who had problems before the procedure.

- **Hysterectomy makes you put on weight.** Again, yes and no. Weight gain is not caused by hysterectomy but by an inactive lifestyle following the procedure. If you want to prevent weight gain, you will, by resuming physical activity as soon as possible after surgery.

What Happens Next?

There are many factors to consider when trying to decide between medication alone, hysterectomy, or another alternative technique. The decision may ultimately depend on the severity of your condition and your symptoms. If you are having trouble deciding, seek a second opinion from another physician who is knowledgeable about your condition and the range of procedures available and don't be afraid to ask about his or her experience in performing the procedure you're interested in. Do not be embarrassed to do this because, in the end, you will be the one undergoing the hysterectomy, not your physician. Remember—you are the customer shopping for a service.

Chapter 4

getting ready for your hysterectomy

What Happens in this Chapter

- Planning time off
- Pre-admission tests and procedures
- Consent
- Blood transfusions
- Asking questions

Although waiting for surgery can be stressful, there are things you can do to feel more prepared for your operation. Aside from routine pre-admission tests and procedures, you can take the time to read up on your hysterectomy so that you know exactly what will happen before, during, and after your surgery. You can also organize your recovery time and write down any questions you may wish to ask before you sign the consent form.

Pre-Operative Tests

BEFORE YOUR OPERATION, THERE ARE SPECIFIC TESTS THAT YOU MUST have to determine that you are ready for surgery. Although it can seem a bit overwhelming to undergo a battery of tests, they are routine and will help your operation go smoothly. Your doctors want to make sure that you are as healthy as possible before your hysterectomy.

[S E L F - H E L P]

Relax!

It's normal to feel nervous while waiting for your surgery. See Chapter 10 for some advice on relaxation techniques you might like to try.

"If you're the one that does all the housekeeping, you'll need a bit of a break when you get home. Even if it's minimally invasive the whole episode leaves you tired—takes a little bit of the goodness out of you."

Anne

In most hospitals, you will be seen in the **pre-admission clinic** a few days before your scheduled surgery for a small number of blood tests. These blood tests assess how well your kidneys and liver are working, and whether you are anemic. Your blood may also be cross-matched, so that appropriate blood products can be available in case you need a blood transfusion. It is possible that you will need a transfusion if you are having cancer surgery or you are severely anemic.

If you are under 50 years old, you may also be given a pregnancy test. If you are over 40 years of age, your heart may be checked out with an **ECG** (see Glossary), and if you are a heavy smoker, asthmatic, or at risk for lung disease you will get a chest X-ray to make sure that your heart and lungs are healthy. An abnormality in your heart or lungs could complicate your anesthesia and post-operative recovery.

Pre-Hysterectomy Arrangements

We know, you're superwoman, but now it's time to let someone else do the work. You'll need to plan plenty of recovery time and you will definitely need some extra help for the first few weeks after your operation. You will not be able to do housework for a while, so leave it to somebody else for about 4 weeks. It's also a good idea to stock up the freezer and get family members organized to take over the cooking for a few weeks. Buy a new robe or pajamas to wear around the house afterward as a visual signal to your family that you need help and rest. You may also want to suspend your gym membership or other sport activities for the 2 months after your procedure.

If you work outside of the home, the amount of time you will need off for your hysterectomy depends on the type of hysterectomy you have and how physically demanding your job is, and how fit you are before surgery.

If you are having a vaginal or laparoscopic hysterectomy, it is best to plan to take about 4 weeks off work. If you are

"Have a bit of a situation set up so by the time you get home for the first week or so things can run somewhat automatically. If you've got small children, you should probably get some help. You deserve a break."

Anne

Back on the Job

You should not drive for 2 weeks after your hysterectomy, so this may affect how early you can return to work.

	Physically Demanding Occupation—At Least:	Sedentary Occupation
Laparoscopic	4-6 weeks off work	2 to 4 weeks off work
Abdominal	6-8 weeks off work	4 to 6 weeks off work
Vaginal	4-6 weeks off work	2 to 4 weeks off work

having abdominal hysterectomy, you will need about 6 weeks off. If your job is fairly sedentary, it may be safe for you to return to work in as little as 4 weeks if you've had abdominal hysterectomy, and 2 weeks if you've had vaginal or laparoscopic hysterectomy. See the Self-Help box for a quick reference on how much time you'll need to take off work. Taking this time is important because it lets you recover fully from the anesthesia and encourages your wounds to heal quickly. By the time you are ready to go back to work, the skin sutures will have been removed or will have disintegrated if dissolving sutures are used.

Some patients like to tidy up their paperwork at home before coming to the hospital for their hysterectomy. Sorting out financial loose ends and updating your will are some suggestions. You may also want to draw up a **living will**. A living will clearly informs your family and your doctor exactly what you would like, and, probably more importantly, would not like, in case of an emergency. These kinds of preparations give many people a sense of comfort. While they may or may not be right for you, they are worth considering.

Consent

Before you have your hysterectomy, you will need to give your **written consent**. This is one of the most important steps of your hysterectomy experience.

What Exactly Is "Consent"?

You make decisions to take risks every day of your life. Some kind of risk is involved when you cross a road, place a bet on a horse, drive your car, or board an airplane. However, when you go into the hospital to have surgery, the risk you take feels different because you are allowing somebody else, usually a doctor, to make decisions for you. Nonetheless, this is a risk just like many others in your life.

Although the doctor will be acting in your best interests, it is still important that you understand exactly what you are giving your permission for, or consent to. You are therefore entitled to know what is going to happen to you, why the procedure is needed, and what the risks and alternatives are.

You may be asked for consent for your hysterectomy as soon as you agree to have the operation, in a pre-admission clinic, or on the day of your procedure. It is important that you read the consent form and understand what it is you are signing. Take a few moments to read through it and, if there is enough time, you can take the form home and take it with you on the day of your procedure. It may be helpful to bring a friend or family member with you to help listen to explanations. It is often difficult to digest everything the doctor is saying. If you are worried about any part of the procedure, or you feel you have not received a clear answer on something, now is the time to say so.

Blood Transfusions

The chances of requiring a blood transfusion during your surgery have been dramatically reduced in recent years. If your physicians think you might need a blood transfusion, they will carefully consider its risks and benefits. The following are important principles of blood conservation, some of which need to be planned a few weeks in advance.

Why Is a Transfusion Needed?

If you lose too much blood (around 2 liters, 2 quarts, or more) during your surgery, your hemoglobin level will fall and your body tissues won't be able to get enough oxygen. This is called anemia (see page 39) and can lead to fatigue, a slow recovery, and impaired healing. A transfusion of blood products such as red cells, can help to prevent this.

How Risky Is a Blood Transfusion?

A blood transfusion has never been safer. Blood is collected from healthy volunteers and tested for a wide range of viruses, including hepatitis B and C, and HIV. The risk of becoming infected with one of these viruses is now quite small (see Key Point box on page 70).

Just for Partners

It's normal for partners of hysterectomy patients to experience feelings that range from anxiety surrounding the dangers of the procedure, to relief that symptoms such as heavy bleeding and cancer may be eliminated after surgery. Some feel helpless because there's no quick fix for the problem and worry that their partner's hysterectomy will affect their sex life. Dealing with menopausal symptoms that accompany removal of the ovaries is also challenging for many partners. Lesbian partners may even feel guilty that they aren't the ones who need a hysterectomy and male partners sometimes worry about catching their partner's cancer.

The best way to deal with these fears is to discuss them with your partner and her doctor before the procedure. Feel free to accompany her to medical appointments and make sure all of your questions are answered. After the surgery, continue an open line of communication so that you can decide together on the best time to resume your sex life and deal with any difficulties if they arise.

Other common risks of blood transfusions are fever and itchiness, which occur in around 1 in 100 people and are easily treated. Rejection (**hemolytic**) reactions, caused by the incompatibility of the two blood types, can also occur in around 1 in 12,000 people. These are mostly prevented by a special blood test called **cross-matching** before your surgery.

What Are Your Chances of a Transfusion?

Only about 1 to 2 percent of patients (up to 1 in 50) undergoing a simple hysterectomy need a blood transfusion after surgery. However, patients undergoing more extensive operations usually lose more blood and are therefore more likely to need a transfusion. The single most important factor in needing a transfusion after surgery is anemia before surgery. This is one of the reasons your blood is tested before your hysterectomy, so that you and your physician can correct your anemia before you have your procedure.

Blood Conservation Strategies

Spotting and Treating Anemia

Treating anemia before surgery is one of the most important things you and your physician can do to reduce the chances of a blood transfusion. If your blood tests before surgery show that your hemoglobin is low, your physician may prescribe iron tablets, vitamins (e.g., B12 or folate), or injections of a hormone called erythropoietin. Erythropoietin is naturally secreted by the kidneys to stimulate the body to make more red blood cells and a synthetic version (epoetin alfa) will gradually correct your anemia by increasing the number of red blood cells in your body. You may also be given one of several hormonal agents to prevent you from doing any further bleeding until your surgery. That way, you have a chance to replenish what you have lost.

[**KEY POINT**]

Donor blood transfusions are potentially life-saving and have never been safer. The risk of HIV infection from donated blood in the U.S. is now almost 1 in 2 million. The risk of hepatitis B infection is around 1 in 140,000. By comparison, your risk of dying in a motor vehicle accident is around 1 in 10,000.

Blood Banking

One of the best-known blood conservation strategies is blood banking or **autologous blood donation (ABD)**. This involves coming to the clinic several times before your surgery to donate I unit of blood each time. Your blood is stored in the blood bank, reserved for your use, for up to 42 days. If your stored blood is not used by you, it is discarded.

You should talk to your physician at least 3 weeks before your surgery if you are interested in blood banking, but bear in mind it may not be available at your hospital or your surgeon may not recommend it for your operation because your risk of a blood transfusion may be very low. Obviously, ABD is not an option if you need surgery urgently.

While pre-donating blood may seem an attractive option, it does have a number of disadvantages, and you and your physician should weigh these carefully against its benefits. Despite careful storage and handling of your pre-donated blood, it will not be exactly the same when you receive it back because of chemical changes during storage. Your pre-donated blood may even become infected with bacteria that will be passed on to you. There is also the small risk of clerical error, so you may end up receiving the wrong blood. The most important downside to pre-donation is that taking your own blood from you may actually make you anemic before surgery. One in 10 people who pre-donate go on to have a blood transfusion, either of their own blood or from the donor pool.

Planning Ahead

You should ask your surgeon, anesthesiologist, or both, about your blood conservation options as soon as you know that you are having surgery. If you are anemic, remember that taking your iron tablets as prescribed and eating an iron-rich diet may help stave off a blood transfusion. Iron-rich foods include organ meats, turkey and chicken (dark meat), dried fruits, whole grain cereals, peas, beans, and dark green, leafy vegetables (e.g., spinach). You can obtain reliable information on blood conservation from the American Association of Blood Banks (www.aabb.org) and the American Red Cross (www.redcross.org).

Asking Questions

Asking questions is an important part of your surgery experience. You have the right to fully understand what will happen to your body, and you should feel free to ask any questions you like before signing the consent form. If you can't get the answers you need, you can postpone giving your consent until you are sure that having a hysterectomy is right for you. Reading up on hysterectomy beforehand is helpful because you will understand more of what you are being told and be able to come up with questions more easily. It is sometimes helpful to write down your questions so that you don't forget them; patients often remember their questions after they leave the doctor's office.

Questions You Could Ask Before Your Hysterectomy

- ○ Why do I need a hysterectomy?
- ○ What are my other options?
- ○ What could happen if I choose not to have a hysterectomy?
- ○ How urgent is my surgery?
- ○ What kind of anesthetic will I have?
- ○ How many incisions will there be and where?
- ○ What will you take out?
- ○ What are the differences between abdominal, vaginal, and laparoscopic hysterectomy?
- ○ What are the risks and benefits of each of these procedures?
- ○ Are all of these procedures available to me?
- ○ Should my cervix be removed?
- ○ What are the risks and benefits of not removing my cervix?
- ○ Are you going to remove my ovaries?
- ○ Will a hysterectomy affect my sex life?
- ○ If I have a hysterectomy laparoscopically or vaginally, how is it possible for my uterus to be removed through the small incision?
- ○ How can I reduce my risk of a blood transfusion?
- ○ Will my appearance change after my hysterectomy?
- ○ What medications, such as hormonal replacements, will I have to take after my surgery?

The Night Before

The day before your operation, you should not eat or drink after midnight. If your surgery is expected to be more extensive, you might be instructed to have a bowel-prep the day before surgery. While a bowel-prep may sound unpleasant, it is really very straightforward.

1. Beginning at noon the day before surgery, you will be asked to stop eating solid food and consume only clear fluids, such as broth, juice, Jell-O, water, or tea.

2. At about 2:00 p.m., you will be asked to drink two vials of a laxative called Phospha-soda that you get by prescription from a pharmacy. This laxative will encourage a bowel movement.

You may also be prescribed an antibiotic and an enema the evening before your hysterectomy, both of which may be particularly important if you have had other abdominal operations, because your bowel is more at risk for injury. The purpose of the antibiotic-enema combination is to clean and empty your intestines in case they are accidentally injured during the operation. A cleaner intestinal environment means that the surgeon will be able to make repairs with minimal complications.

What Happens Next?

Once you have signed the consent form, the next step is the hysterectomy procedure itself.

Chapter 5

the day of your hysterectomy

What Happens in this Chapter

- Making a hospital checklist
- Arrival at the hospital
- Tips for friends and family
- Medications you may be given
- Transfer to the operating room

The day of your surgery finally arrives. It is normal for you to feel anxious before having your hysterectomy, but knowing what will happen can help you to feel more relaxed and in control. You may be hospitalized the morning of your surgery or the day before. When you get to the hospital you will be assigned a bed and a nurse will look after you. There will be some routine tests and you will then be taken to the operating room where your hysterectomy will be performed.

Planning Your Day

MANY PATIENTS FIND THAT STAYING ORGANIZED HELPS TO RELIEVE some of their stress. Below is a hospital checklist so that you won't forget anything when you're planning for your hospital stay. Because you may be in the hospital for several days, be sure to pack toiletries and something to help pass the time, such as a good book, crossword puzzles, magazines, or knitting. You may also be able to watch television when you arrive. These kinds of distractions are particularly helpful while you are waiting for your surgery to begin. Be sure to bring a list of medications that you normally take, and remember to make arrangements to be driven home from the hospital when it's time to leave because you will be advised not to drive yourself.

> "My advice would be, to keep busy, watch a video or read a book and not sit around worrying about things."
>
> **Dawn**

Hospital Checklist

The hospital is a busy place. Your care team won't necessarily have the time or resources to provide you with everything you need during your hospital stay. There are a number of items that you should bring with you to the hospital and some that you should leave at home. Use this checklist to help you prepare for your hospital stay:

DO NOT...

- eat or drink (even water) after midnight. If you normally take medications that require you to drink water, inform the doctor or the nurse well in advance of your operation. You may brush your teeth, but spit the water out.

- shave your abdomen unless you are instructed otherwise. Studies have shown that incisions on shaved areas tend to become infected.

- bring valuables such as jewelry, watches, credit cards, laptops, cell phones, and large amounts of money to the hospital. Unfortunately, there have been situations in every hospital where items have been misplaced, lost, or even stolen.

- bring work with you. You will need to rest and heal while you are in the hospital.

DO...

- bring a full list of your medications.

- pack some reading material with you to help pass the time before your surgery. However, the sedative medication used during your procedure will leave you feeling drowsy afterward, so you might have trouble concentrating.

- pack personal items, such as toiletries, pyjamas, a robe, and slippers. You may even want to bring your own pillow and pillowcase, which can help you rest more easily.

- pack attractive, but comfortable clothes for when you leave the hospital.

- bring a list of questions, or a pen and paper to write down any that you think of at the last minute.

- bring someone for emotional support.

- remember to bring this book!

Hospital Arrival

Just as you have carefully prepared for your hospital visit, the hospital staff is prepared to care for you. When you arrive at the hospital, you will be assigned a room and a nurse who will look after you (along with several other patients). Feel free to talk to your nurse about any last-minute concerns that you might have. He or she will ask you to change into a hospital gown, and you will be given an identification bracelet that has your name, your physician's name, and the name of any medication allergies you have on it. The nurse will ask you questions about your health and make sure that you fully understand your surgery. An intravenous line is then inserted into one of your arms. This line will be used to give you fluids, and administer drugs during and after your hysterectomy. You will not be allowed to drink until after your procedure.

If you have not had a recent physical examination, often a physician will perform one. Routine blood tests, an ECG, and a chest X-ray (if you are at risk for lung disease) may be performed if they have not yet been done. You will also have a chance to talk to the anesthesiologist who will be in charge of your anesthetic and pain management during and after your hysterectomy. You will then give your consent for the operation if you have not already done so.

Medications Before Your Procedure

Sedatives

It is normal to feel anxious before your hysterectomy. Mild oral sedatives or sleeping pills given the night before surgery will help you relax and get a good night's sleep. If you're still nervous when

Self-Help on the Day

- Ask questions *before* you go into the operating room for your hysterectomy.

- Before going to the operating room, give the following items to a friend or family member for safekeeping: hair clips, hairpiece or wig, contact lenses, jewelry, eyeglasses, hearing aids, dentures, and other prostheses.

- Makeup may be smudged during surgery but if you feel better wearing it, then leave it on except for mascara, which could scratch your eyes.

- Underwear should normally be removed as well. If you have your period, ask your nurse for disposable panties for use with a sanitary pad, or use a tampon.

you reach the hospital, the anesthesiologist may give you a fast-acting sedative. This sedative will make you drowsy, but you will still be conscious because your medical team will need to talk to you. They want you to be as comfortable as possible throughout your surgery experience.

Antibiotics

You may be given prophylactic (preventive) antibiotics prior to your surgery. This is especially important if you have a history of rheumatic heart disease or have a heart murmur. Even if you don't have a heart condition, prophylactic antibiotics are usually administered before a hysterectomy in order to prevent infection.

Blood Thinners

If you have a history of blood clots in your legs or lungs, you will need an injection of a blood-thinning medication (anticoagulant) called heparin. Heparin ensures that your blood does not clot inside your blood vessels. If your blood clots, your blood vessels could become blocked, or a clot could travel into your lungs or heart and cause problems. However, one complication of blood thinners is that they can make you bleed more during surgery. Your doctor might also prescribe stockings that you will wear during surgery to enhance the circulation of your blood.

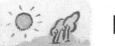

[KEY POINT]

You should inform your doctor before your operation if you regularly take a weak blood thinner, such as ASA (e.g., Aspirin). If you are on a more powerful blood thinner, such as warfarin (e.g., Coumadin), your doctor will advise you to stop taking it about 3 days before your hysterectomy. Instead, you will be given a heparin injection.

Transfer to the Operating Room

Your physician can only estimate what time your surgery will take place, unless your operation is scheduled to be the first one of the day. The length of other surgeries and unexpected emergencies will influence when your operation can begin.

Friends and Family

Depending on your hospital's policy, friends and family members may be allowed to stay with you in the hospital ward. Their presence often helps to relieve anxiety, and they can provide you with support when you are giving your consent or asking questions. You may want to have the support of your sexual partner so that both of you can learn together about the procedure and your recovery. It is important that both you and your partner understand that a hysterectomy does not necessarily have the negative psychological and sexual effects that many people think it does.

> "I had great confidence in my doctor and he was there for me, and that makes a big difference. I trusted him and I knew I was in good hands. I now feel great."
>
> **Betty**

Friends and family will not be allowed to stay with you after your transfer to the operating room. There is usually a waiting area for them if they wish to stay in the hospital during your operation. If your friends and family do not want to stay in the waiting area, they should leave details of how they can they be reached in the unlikely event that a member of the surgical team wishes to speak with them during your surgery. Most surgeons also like to talk to family or friends after the operation to explain the outcome of the surgery.

Your hysterectomy will take 1 to 3 hours depending on when the surgery started and how complicated it is. Following your hysterectomy, you will be transferred to the recovery room or **post-anesthesia care unit (PACU)** where a team of nurses will look after you. Once you are stable and more alert—usually after 2 to 3 hours—you will be transferred back to your hospital room, and your friends and family will be able to visit you.

What Happens Next?

Once you are in the operating room, your hysterectomy procedure will begin.

Chapter 6

the hysterectomy procedure

What Happens in this Chapter

- A step-by-step guide to your hysterectomy
- Abdominal, vaginal, and laparoscopic hysterectomy
- The general anesthetic
- Regional anesthesia
- Tests and investigations during the operation
- Other procedures
- Closing the incision

Hysterectomy is a procedure to remove the uterus and it can be done in several different ways. The traditional route—a direct incision in the abdomen—is now being replaced by vaginal or laparoscopic hysterectomy in some women. There's also a choice of what comes out and what stays in. Depending on the reason for the surgery, the cervix or ovaries may be left in place or removed along with the uterus. Whatever the route or whatever surgery you have, your hysterectomy will probably take about 2 hours, after which you will go back to the recovery room.

What Is Hysterectomy?

A HYSTERECTOMY IS A SURGICAL PROCEDURE TO REMOVE THE uterus. It is an essential procedure for women with invasive cancer of the uterus, cervix, vagina, ovaries, or fallopian tubes. It is also necessary to treat life-threatening bleeding, severe pelvic inflammatory disease that does not respond to other treatment, and complications of pregnancy such as rupture of the uterus. It is also the treatment of choice for large fibroids that are causing heavy bleeding and severely affecting quality of life.

For all other conditions, including endometriosis (page 19), pelvic pain, premenstrual syndrome, endometrial hyperplasia (page 18), uterine prolapse (page 24), smaller, less annoying fibroids, and a variety of other gynecological conditions, hysterectomy is an option—but only one option. Never be forced into a hysterectomy for these conditions. Chapter 3 covers a full discussion of whether hysterectomy is right for you.

As with all surgical procedures, there are several different ways to perform hysterectomy. Depending on your own condition and the facilities available locally, you may be able to choose the type of surgery you want. Your surgeon should be able to advise you what is available.

What Is Removed?

The types of hysterectomy are shown in Figure 6–1. A hysterectomy can involve removal of the entire uterus (total hysterectomy) or the cervix may be left in (subtotal or partial hysterectomy). When the ovaries and fallopian tubes are also removed the procedure is called salpingo-oophorectomy. If you have invasive cancer, you will probably need a radical hysterectomy, in which the top of the vagina is removed as well as the uterus, and usually the fallopian tubes, and ovaries. The pros and cons of these different procedures are discussed fully in Chapter 3. In the present chapter, we will concentrate on how each procedure is carried out.

Figure 6–1. Types of Hysterectomy

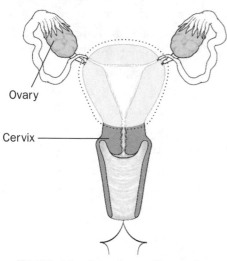

Ovary

Cervix

(A) Subtotal hysterectomy. The body of the uterus is removed, but the cervix remains in place.

(B) Total hysterectomy. The entire uterus, including the cervix, is removed.

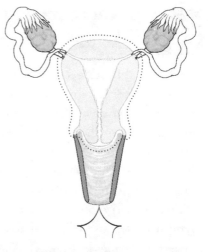

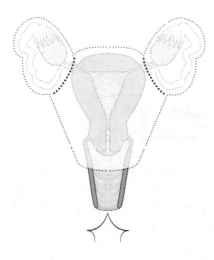

(C) Radical hysterectomy. The entire uterus and the top portion of the vagina are removed along with the tissues surrounding the uterus and cervix. The ovaries and the fallopian tubes may also be removed, a procedure called **radical hysterectomy with salpingo-oophorectomy**.

Surgical Choices

In addition to the choices of what comes out and what stays in, there are also three main ways to perform hysterectomy: abdominal hysterectomy, laparoscopic hysterectomy, and vaginal hysterectomy. Gynecological surgeons tend to specialize in one or another of them. While this is a good thing—they get really good at their own particular technique—it can sometimes mean that a physician will recommend one procedure over another just because he or she is better at it. Again, your own situation may mean that choice is not possible, but if you do have a choice, make sure you choose your surgeon according to the technique you want, not vice versa. Again, Chapter 3 discusses how you should make your choice, while the present chapter will concentrate on the practicalities.

Abdominal Hysterectomy

Abdominal hysterectomy or **laparotomy** is still the most common type of hysterectomy. This traditional approach involves making an incision in your abdomen 12 to 15 cm (4 to 6 inches) long, either vertically from the navel to below the pubic hairline, or horizontally above the pubic hair—a **Pfannenstiel** or **bikini incision** (see Figure 6–2). An abdominal incision may be the only route out for a very large, bulky uterus. It is also particularly important for cancers, or where the surgeon has other good reasons for needing access to lymph nodes and other structures in your abdomen.

Laparoscopic Hysterectomy

Today, many hysterectomies can be done by this technique, which involves using a surgical telescope (laparoscope) to look inside the abdomen and examine the internal organs via a small incision below the navel (see Figure 6–3). The camera is connected to a TV

Figure 6–2. Incisions for Hysterectomy

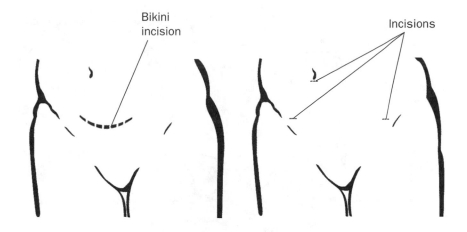

Bikini incision

Incisions

(A) For an abdominal hysterectomy, a single "bikini incision" is made just above the pubic hair.

(B) A laparoscopic hysterectomy requires three or four small incisions.

monitor, and the surgeon operates by viewing the monitor. There are usually two monitors, one for the surgeon and one for his or her assistant.

Laparoscopic hysterectomy involves making three or four small incisions between 0.5 and 2 cm long (1/4 to 3/4 inch) in the abdomen: one small incision below the navel, two more incisions on each side of the

> "With this minimally invasive stuff you're off home the next day and you're told, don't worry it's minimal, minimal. Well, it's not so minimal. You've got a couple of puncture wounds, you've had an anesthetic, you've been given drugs. Inside, you're uncomfortable and you're sore and it takes time to get over that. They'll manage, but if they think they're going to wake up and it will be like nothing has happened, that's not always true."
>
> **Anne**

Figure 6–3. Laparoscopy

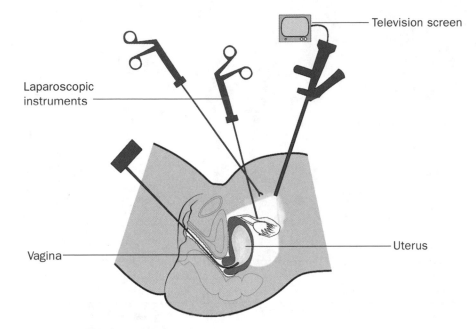

Television screen

Laparoscopic instruments

Vagina

Uterus

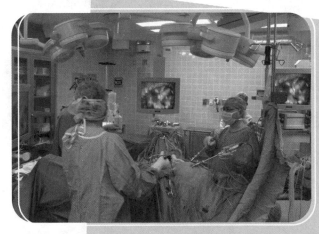

A laparoscopic hysterectomy is performed using long, thin instruments inserted through small incisions in your abdomen. One of the instruments contains a tiny camera. The surgeon operates by watching the procedure on a television screen. Laparoscopy can also be used for diagnosis.

abdomen, and occasionally another incision of 0.5 cm (¼ inch) in the middle of the pubic hairline.

Once the incisions are made, carbon dioxide will be introduced into your abdomen, just like blowing up a balloon. This is necessary in order to see your pelvic organs clearly. After your hysterectomy your body will absorb the excess gas. Although carbon dioxide itself is harmless, you may get shoulder pains for a day or two after the procedure due to the gas stimulating the diaphragm (a muscle that forms the floor of the chest). Because gas goes upward, you will feel the shoulder pain when you are standing or sitting.

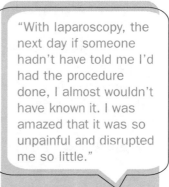

"With laparoscopy, the next day if someone hadn't have told me I'd had the procedure done, I almost wouldn't have known it. I was amazed that it was so unpainful and disrupted me so little."

Dawn

Once your abdomen is full of gas, the surgical team will insert three or four long metal tubes called **trocars**. The trocars, which have valves at one end, stay in place during the procedure and allow the laparoscope and surgical instruments to be moved in and out of the abdomen and changed as needed.

Laparoscopic instruments such as forceps and scissors are very long (around 40 cm or 15 inches) and thin (less than 1 cm or ½ inch in diameter) so that they can fit down the trocars.

Compared to abdominal hysterectomy, the hospital stay and recovery are shorter with laparoscopic hysterectomy. However, the procedure is not possible for all women. Chapter 3 weighs the risks and benefits of this approach.

Vaginal Hysterectomy

In vaginal hysterectomy, you do not need a cut in your abdomen. Instead, the uterus is removed through the "natural passage"—i.e., the vagina. In order to do this, an incision is made around the cervix at the top of the vagina and the uterus is removed through this incision (see Figure 6–4). The top of the vagina is then closed.

Vaginal hysterectomy is particularly useful for women whose uterus is sagging into the vagina, a condition called uterine prolapse (see page 24). Although the advantage of this technique is that there is no visible scar on the abdomen, the vaginal route may not be possible if there are very large fibroids or if it is important to be able to see other organs high in the pelvis. Furthermore, the ovaries might not be reachable.

A combined laparoscopic and vaginal hysterectomy is called **laparoscopic-assisted vaginal hysterectomy**. In this procedure, part of the operation is done by laparoscopy, then the uterus is removed through the vagina.

Figure 6–4. Vaginal Hysterectomy

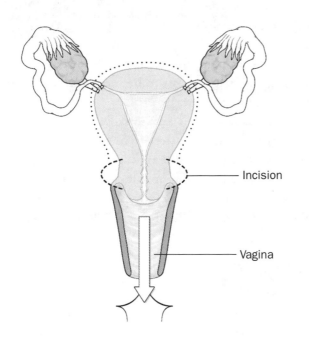

Incision

Vagina

In this type of hysterectomy, an incision is made in the top of the vagina, and the whole uterus (including the cervix) is removed through the vagina.

Getting Ready

Inside the operating room, you will be asked to lie down on the operating table. Your arms will be extended and placed on arm boards. Unless you have an intravenous line already, the anesthesiologist will insert one, numbing the area first with local anesthesic.

At this point, one of the operating room nurses will apply a ground pad—a sticky pad—on your thigh. This safety precaution is needed because an **electrosurgery device** will be used to seal your blood vessels during the procedure. A small plastic sleeve will also be slipped onto one of your fingers to monitor your blood-oxygen level during surgery. The team will also fit an automatic blood pressure cuff on your upper arm to measure your blood pressure continuously during surgery. You will feel a "squeezing" on and off while your blood pressure is automatically taken. Three sticky electrodes that monitor your heart activity will also be attached to your chest. When the monitors and lines are in place, you are ready for your anesthetic.

The General Anesthetic

Some people prefer to be "out cold" for surgery. This is called a general anesthetic.

A general anesthetic is not one drug, but a cocktail of medications—each with different roles. It includes drugs to put you to sleep (induction drugs), vapor drugs to keep you asleep, and muscle relaxants. The medication to make you sleep is given through your I.V. while you breathe oxygen through a mask. From the time a general anesthetic starts, patients rarely have any recall of events and 70 percent of patients do not remember entering the operating room. Your anesthesiologist can precisely control your

The Oxygen Mask

The oxygen mask often has a plastic (beach ball-like) smell, or it may be scented to cover this odor. Be assured that, unless your anesthesiologist tells you otherwise, the strange smell is not the anesthetic vapor. You will receive your general anesthetic through your I.V. line.

level of consciousness and will take you from being wide-awake to deep surgical anesthesia in a matter of moments.

The risks of general anesthesia are carefully managed using an array of sophisticated monitors and your anesthesiologist will watch you carefully throughout the surgery. The dangers of a general anesthetic are now just a small part of the overall risks of surgery. Once you are asleep, the anesthesiologist will insert a plastic tube called an **endotracheal tube** into your mouth and trachea (windpipe). Oxygen and anesthetic gas will be delivered into your lungs through this tube. You may also receive a **nasogastric tube** through your nose to your stomach to suck any fluid or gas. This makes the stomach smaller and surgery easier, especially laparoscopic surgery.

How Do They Know I'm Asleep?

[MORE DETAIL]

Many people fear that they might wake up or be aware during surgery. This is very rare and happens in fewer than three in 1000 operations. When it does happen, most patients describe the memory as brief, vague and painless.

Regional Anesthesia

The other type of anesthesia that can be used is regional anesthesia, or a "block." There are two types of block. For a **spinal anesthetic**, a very tiny needle is placed through your back into the spinal canal. A small amount of local anesthesia is added to the fluid bathing the nerves in your back making you numb from about the waist down in 2-5 minutes. For an **epidural anesthetic**, a larger volume of local anesthetic solution is injected into the space surrounding the spinal canal, and therefore more gradually causes numbness. Medication can be given through your I.V. to make you as groggy as you would like to be, once the block is working.

Final Preparations

A tube (catheter) is inserted into your bladder to keep it empty during the hysterectomy. This makes the operation easier as a full bladder interferes with the surgery and increases the risk of bladder injury.

For vaginal and laparoscopic hysterectomy, you will be placed in the **lithotomy position**, in which your legs rest on two platforms called **stirrups** and your knees are bent at about a 20-degree angle and spread apart. This gives the gynecologic surgeon and his or her assistants good access to the surgical site. For abdominal hysterectomy, you will lie flat on your back. If you have back problems be sure to alert your nurse. Pillows can be placed

> "My doctor was really surprised because he didn't expect what he found. My uterus was bigger than he had anticipated so apparently I was under a bit longer than he thought I would be."
>
> **Betty**

Your Hysterectomy Step by Step

[**MORE DETAIL**]

The following are the basic steps of your hysterectomy. If this is all the detail you want or need to know, feel free to skip to Chapter 8.

1. The monitors are connected to you, e.g., blood pressure cuff, chest electrodes.
2. An intravenous line is put in your arm for medications and fluids.
3. An oxygen mask is placed over your mouth and nose and you are asked to breathe normally.
4. You are given a general anesthetic through the intravenous line.
5. Once you are asleep, you are attached to a breathing machine (ventilator).
6. You are placed in the correct position for the procedure and washed with antiseptic.
7. The incisions are made—one incision in your abdomen if you are having an abdominal hysterectomy, three or four small incisions in your abdomen for a laparoscopy, or one incision in your vagina for a vaginal hysterectomy.
8. The uterus is separated from the surrounding tissues and organs.
9. The uterus (and in some procedures, the fallopian tubes and ovaries) is removed.
10. The surgeon checks the organs in your abdomen for any abnormalities.
11. A sample of fluid from the abdomen and any suspicious-looking tissue is sent to the laboratory.
12. Other procedures are carried out as needed (e.g., vaginal repairs).
13. The incisions are closed.
14. You leave the operating room still groggy but usually breathing on your own.

under your knees and you should be positioned for surgery while you are still awake to ensure that the position is comfortable.

Finally, one of the surgical team will wash your body and vagina with an antiseptic solution to reduce the risk of infection. The surgery can now be started.

The Hysterectomy Procedure

The first step is to detach the uterus from all its supporting tissues and ligaments. The bladder, which is normally attached to the cervix, is then carefully separated from the uterus down to the level of the upper vagina. This allows the uterus to be removed without risking injury to the bladder or **ureter**, the tube that drains urine from the kidney to the bladder. You may be given a dye through the I.V. that colors your urine so your surgeon can be sure that no injury to the urinary tract has occurred.

If the ovaries and fallopian tubes are staying put, the ligaments between them and the uterus are also carefully detached. Otherwise, they will be left in place.

The uterus is now only attached to the cervix and fallopian tubes. If you are having a total hysterectomy, the next stage is to separate the cervix from the vagina. If you are having subtotal hysterectomy, the separation will take place along an imaginary line between the cervix and the body of the uterus. If your fallopian tubes are to be left intact, they will also be separated from the uterus at this point.

The uterus is now free in the abdominal cavity and can be removed. In abdominal hysterectomy, the whole uterus is carefully lifted through the incision. In laparoscopic hysterectomy, the uterus will be removed piece by piece, unless the cervix is also being removed, in which case the whole uterus is extracted out through the vagina. If you are having vaginal hysterectomy, your uterus will be removed through the incision in the vaginal wall, either whole or piece by piece.

An important aspect of hysterectomy is minimizing the risk of bleeding. Blood vessels are usually tied with sutures that dissolve in 4 to 6 weeks, although increasingly in vaginal and laparoscopic hysterectomy, surgeons prefer to seal the blood vessels with a variety of devices.

Extra Procedures

Exploration
Although the main goal of your surgery is hysterectomy, your gynecologic surgeon will also take the opportunity to do a thorough examination of the inside of your abdomen. With abdominal hysterectomy, the surgeon cannot see the organs in the upper abdomen such as the liver, spleen, and stomach, and he or she will examine these organs by feeling them with his or her hands. With laparoscopy, the lens of the laparoscope is inside the abdomen and all the abdominal organs can be clearly seen. If the organs do not look or feel normal, a biopsy or a consultation with another specialist is done. With a vaginal incision, such exploration of the upper abdomen is not possible.

Peritoneal Fluid Test
If you are having surgery for cancer or suspected cancer, the fluid in your abdomen will be sampled and sent to the laboratory for microscopic examination. To get enough fluid for the test, the surgeon may rinse your abdominal organs with a small amount of sterile fluid first.

Urethral Suspension Surgery
This procedure is designed to help women who have severe **stress urinary incontinence**, in which they lose a small amount of urine

every time they cough, sneeze, or strain. **Urethral suspension surgery**, which can be done at the time of hysterectomy, involves supporting the urethra, the tube the runs from your bladder to the outside, and strengthening its supporting tissue.

AP Repair

If the uterus is sagging into the vagina, the bladder and rectum are often dragged down with it. **AP repair (anterior and posterior colporraphy)** involves restoring the bladder and the rectum to their rightful places. It is performed toward the end of a vaginal hysterectomy.

Node Removal

If you are having surgery for cancer, the surgeon may also remove the lymph nodes inside your abdomen. **Lymph nodes** are grape-like structures that act as a filter to the spread of infection and, to a certain extent, cancer. All body fluids drain through the lymph nodes, so if cancer cells have started to spread out from the affected organ, they will sometimes lodge in the nodes.

Laboratory analysis of the nodes will tell you whether the cancer is still confined to the organs or has spread to the nodes. If this is the case, you may need additional treatment such as chemotherapy or radiation.

Pathological Examination

Any tissue removed at surgery is sent to the laboratory, where it is sliced in many pieces, stained, and then examined under a microscope. The **pathologist**—a doctor whose specialty is diagnosing a disease using laboratory techniques—will be able to tell whether the tissue is normal, contains precancer cells, cancer cells, or other conditions. Depending on the hospital, the results may take a couple of weeks.

Occasionally, if the surgeon sees something suspicious he or she will request a **frozen section** to help him or her decide whether to remove it. For example, a suspicious-looking ovary in a younger woman will create a huge dilemma for a surgeon, who naturally wants to spare the patient early menopause. In this situation, a pathologist will come to the operating room for a consultation and take a small sample of the ovary to the laboratory for immediate processing and microscopic examination. This usually takes about 15 minutes. If definite cancer cells are found, the surgeon will need to go ahead and remove the ovary.

Final Stages

After your hysterectomy is complete, your surgeon will first make sure that there is no internal bleeding and then wash out the inside of your abdomen with a sterile solution to remove any remaining bits of tissue.

Before the incisions are closed, the nurses will re-count all the sponges, needles and other instruments to make sure that nothing is left inside you.

In abdominal hysterectomy, the layer under the skin is closed with sutures that will dissolve in 4 to 6 weeks. You may feel these as little bumps under the skin. The skin incision is then stapled or sutured and covered with a bandage. Unless dissolving sutures are used, these sutures or staples will be removed after about 5 days. You will need to return to the hospital or your doctor's office to have them removed if you are discharged with them still in place.

In laparoscopic hysterectomy, the larger incisions will also have under-skin sutures that gradually dissolve. The top layer of skin, and smaller incisions, will be closed with sutures or taped with adhesive tapes.

After vaginal hysterectomy, the incision in the vagina will be sutured shut and a vaginal pack—a long roll of sponge pressing the vaginal wall—may be inserted into the vagina to reduce the bleeding. This will be removed within 24 to 48 hours.

The catheter in your bladder will often be left in place until you are able to get to the bathroom yourself.

Orders and Reports

Immediately following your hysterectomy, your doctor or the assistant will notify your family and then write a report of the operation, covering what was found and what was done during your hysterectomy. He or she will also write orders that prescribe what the nursing staff should do for you. A detailed report of your hysterectomy will also be prepared for the hospital and your doctor's medical records.

What Happens Next?

Once your operation is finished, you will be wheeled into the recovery room. The anesthesiologist and the operating room nurse will thoroughly brief the recovery room nurses on your procedure. Chapter 8 tells you what to expect as you wake up and begin your recovery.

Chapter 7

alternatives to hysterectomy

What Happens in this Chapter

- The pros and cons of doing nothing
- Tricks to try before you decide on surgery
- Hormone and non-hormone treatments
- Why a D&C should not be your first option
- The facts on uterine fibroid embolization, endometrial ablation, myomectomy, and myolysis

Women can now choose from a wider variety of alternatives to hysterectomy than ever before. Based on your own particular condition, some of these won't be suitable for you, and some simply won't work—or will only provide temporary relief. However, knowledge is power, and understanding the alternatives is always a good thing, even if you ultimately decide that hysterectomy is the right choice.

IN THIS CHAPTER, WE DISCUSS THE MOST COMMON ALTERNATIVES to hysterectomy, along with their advantages and disadvantages. For a more detailed discussion on how to choose between them and hysterectomy, see Chapter 3.

Wait and See

What Is It?

The technical name for this medical option is **watchful waiting** or **close follow-up**. Basically, it means that you and your physician do nothing but keep a close eye on you, which in practice means a gynecological check-up every 6 months. If something changes, or you decide that you need more help, your physician will then spring into action.

This approach is obviously not an option if you have severe hemorrhaging or cancer. It may also be impractical if you have very heavy bleeding that is severely restricting your life. However, it is likely to be the right choice if you have small fibroids discovered during a routine exam and you have no symptoms. Hysterectomy used to be recommended for symptomless fibroids in case they got bigger and more difficult to remove, or turned into cancer (**leiomyosarcoma**). In fact, studies have proven that these concerns are unfounded. Women with medium-sized fibroids have no more problems after surgery than women with small fibroids, and the risk of dying during hysterectomy (1 in 1,000) is much greater than the risk of developing leiomyosarcoma. So don't be persuaded into a hysterectomy "just in case" for symptomless fibroids. If they are not causing problems, leave them alone.

[KEY POINT]

If it isn't broken, don't fix it. Don't be persuaded to have surgery if you have no symptoms unless you have cancer.

Watchful waiting may also work for you if you have abnormal bleeding and/or fibroids and you are in your late forties or early fifties. After menopause, bleeding will stop and your fibroids will shrink anyway, so it may be worth waiting for this to happen. Although menopause is difficult to predict, your doctor can test for the hormone FSH (see page 13) to see if you are close to, or already in, menopause.

You can combine all this watching and waiting with some self-help measures (see Self-Help box), or another non-surgical option such as hormone treatment (see page 105).

"When I first started having problems they put me on the birth control pill. Although I went through a lot of different ones, it did control the bleeding at first and I stayed on it for almost 10 years."

Silvia

Advantages and Disadvantages

The advantage of this watchful waiting is that you are spared an inconvenient and uncomfortable hospital procedure for a while, perhaps forever. It also buys you time to try some self-help measures. The disadvantage is that you may have to continue to put up with your symptoms for a few more years.

Bleeding? Try This First

If you have a gynecological problem, you do not have to go the surgical route right away. Some problems resolve themselves and others are caused by factors that you can change. While you are deciding about surgery try the following:

- **Antiprostaglandins such as mefenamic acid (e.g., Ponstel).** These drugs can reduce bleeding by as much as 30 percent.
- **Get a better painkiller.** There are several good prescription drugs for treating menstrual pain.
- **Stop the pill.** An excess of estrogen may make fibroids grow and can increase bleeding, so if you are taking hormones (HRT or the contraceptive pill), consider stopping them to see if the bleeding improves.
- **Go on the pill.** The contraceptive pill can also relieve some types of irregular or heavy bleeding. If you aren't on it, speak to your doctor about a trial.
- **Ask about other hormone therapies** such as progesterone, or estrogen-blocking drugs.
- **Lose some weight.** Because estrogen is stored in body fat, losing weight may improve your bleeding problems.
- **Are you herbal?** Herbs such as ginseng and cohosh have estrogenic properties—stop using them and see if this helps.
- **Don't forget soy.** Soy also has estrogenic properties (page 165), so if it's a staple in your diet, consider switching to something else for a while and see if your symptoms improve.
- **Stressed out?** High stress levels can make menstrual problems worse. Exercise, relaxation, and massage can all help; see Chapter 10.
- **Scrunch and hold.** Kegel exercises (page 168) can help with uterine prolapse and make a hysterectomy unnecessary.
- **Go organic.** If you eat red meat and dairy products try switching to organic products. Hormones used in conventional animal feed may be affecting you.
- **Use antibiotics correctly.** Before having a hysterectomy for severe pelvic inflammatory disease, make sure your doctor has tried intravenous antibiotics as well as pills.

Non-Hormone Therapy

What Is It?

Effective painkillers for your menstrual pain may be all that you need to keep going until menopause, when your fibroids will shrink and the bleeding stop anyway. The most effective drugs for pain and bleeding are **antiprostaglandins** such as mefenamic acid (e.g., Ponstel), naproxen (e.g., Anaprox, Aleve), ibuprofen (e.g., Advil, Motrin) and meclofenamate (Meclomen). These medications block prostaglandin, a substance that controls menstrual bleeding and pain. Mefenamic acid and meclofenamate also reduce bleeding by as much as 30 percent. Ibuprofen is an effective painkiller, but its effects on bleeding have not been tested. These drugs are best for women whose main symptom is painful and heavy periods.

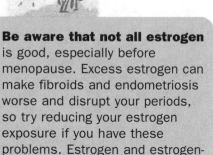

[**KEY POINT**]

Be aware that not all estrogen is good, especially before menopause. Excess estrogen can make fibroids and endometriosis worse and disrupt your periods, so try reducing your estrogen exposure if you have these problems. Estrogen and estrogen-like chemicals are found in red meat, soy, herbs such as ginseng, and the contraceptive pill. Also, drinking alcohol every day can double blood levels of estrogen.

Advantages and Disadvantages

The advantage of antiprostaglandin drugs like mefenamic acid or ibuprofen is that they are easy to take and work well for many women. The disadvantage is that they belong to the same drug class as acetyl-salicylic acid or ASA (e.g., Aspirin) so they can cause stomach problems if taken long term. Mefenamic acid works best if taken a day or so before bleeding and pain starts, so it is best for women with regular cycles.

Hormone Therapy

What Is It?

The activities of your uterus are controlled by hormones, so hormone therapy makes sense. What works best depends on what's wrong.

If your problem is an irregular cycle and heavy bleeding, the combined oral contraceptive pill ("the pill") may help by halting ovulation and thinning out the lining of the uterus. Hormone replacement therapy tablets (HRT, see Chapter 12), which have lower doses of estrogen and progesterone than the pill, may be prescribed instead to regulate your cycle. HRT is less useful for heavy bleeding.

If your heavy bleeding and irregularity is caused by insufficient progesterone, artificial progesterone tablets (e.g., Provera or Prometrium) or a **progesterone-coated intrauterine system** (Mirena) can stabilize your cycle and gradually thin out the lining of the uterus. Progesterone is also effective for endometriosis.

Instead of giving you more hormones, another approach is to reduce your hormone levels. Drugs called **gonadotrophin releasing hormone (GnRH) analogues**, given by injection or nasal spray, stop your ovaries producing estrogen and progesterone and thus "starve" your uterus of hormonal stimulation. This can stop your periods entirely and shrink your fibroids. The

> "I got my period and it never stopped. The blood clots were as big as a hand. It was like an open faucet. My physician had me doing Lupron injections because he wanted to try and save my uterus—he really tried—but it didn't work out."
>
> **Silvia**

maximum effect is seen after 3 months. These drugs are also very effective for endometriosis.

Advantages

The advantage of hormone treatments is their effectiveness in many women. HRT and the pill are simple to take. GnRH analogues are especially useful for shrinking fibroids before myomectomy and some types of endometrial ablation, making the procedure easier and safer.

Disadvantages

The disadvantages of all these therapies are the hormone-related side effects, which are quite common. The pill can cause bloating, breast tenderness, mood swings, and headaches. Women on progesterone complain of nausea and weight gain. Both the pill and HRT increase the risk of thrombosis (blood clots), so they may not be suitable for women who are at risk for cardiovascular disease, such as women who smoke, have a history of heart disease or thrombosis, have high blood pressure, or are overweight. The side effects of HRT are also discussed in Chapter 12.

The downside of GnRH analogues is that they cause menopause-like symptoms, such as hot flashes and vaginal dryness, because the ovaries are no longer producing estrogen. Also, some of them, such as goserelin (Zoladex) and leuprolide (Lupron), need to be injected. They are quite expensive as well. Finally, they cannot be used as a long-term treatment because the lack of estrogen weakens the bones and increases the risk of osteoporosis. Once they are stopped, the fibroids will grow back again.

Medication for Menstrual Problems

[**MORE DETAIL**]

Drug	Type of Treatment	What It's Used For
Non-hormonal Treatments		
Antiprostaglandins such as mefenamic acid (e.g., Ponstel) or ibuprofen (e.g., Advil, Motrin)	capsules/pills	Pain relief, reduces swelling and bleeding
Hormonal Treatments		
Combined estrogen/ progesterone		
Oral contraceptives (e.g., Ortho-Novum, Ortho Tri-cyclen)	pills	Make periods less heavy, more regular
Hormone replacement therapy (HRT)	pills	Makes periods more regular, but may not reduce bleeding if periods regular already
Synthetic progesterones		
Norethindrone (e.g., Aygestin, Ortho Micronor, noresthisterone)	pills	Makes periods less heavy, more regular; relieves endometriosis
Medroxyprogesterone (e.g., Amen, Curretab, Provera)	pills	Makes periods less heavy; relieves endometriosis
GnRH analogues Goserelin (Zoladex) Leuprolide acetate (Lupron) Naferelin (Synarel)	injection injection nasal spray	Relieves endometriosis: shrinks the endometriotic tissue and prevents re-growth

107

Dilation and Curettage (D&C)

What Is It?

A D&C is a treatment for heavy menstrual bleeding that involves removing the uterine lining with a spoon-shaped instrument called a curette or a suction device. See page 38 for a detailed description of this procedure.

Advantages and Disadvantages

D&C used to be the standard treatment for abnormal uterine bleeding, but it has now largely fallen out of favor because it is a "blind" technique. The physician cannot see what he or she is scraping and up to 25 percent of the uterus may be missed. In addition, it is a temporary measure because it only removes the top layer of the endometrium. Endometrial biopsy is a better choice for diagnosis, and hysteroscopy plus endometrial ablation are more effective treatments.

Uterine Fibroid Embolization

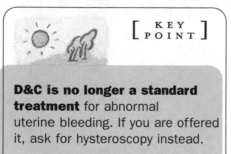

[**KEY POINT**]

D&C is no longer a standard treatment for abnormal uterine bleeding. If you are offered it, ask for hysteroscopy instead.

What Is It?

Uterine fibroid embolization is one of the newest treatments for uterine fibroids without surgery and without a hysterectomy. The goal is to shrink the fibroids and reduce bleeding. It involves blocking the blood supply to the uterus, depriving the fibroids of nutrition.

Uterine fibroid embolization is done by physicians who are skilled in performing procedures under X-ray (**interventional radiologists**). You will be awake but drowsy, under light sedation. First, skin at the area of the groin is injected with local anesthesia to numb the area, then a needle is inserted into a blood vessel called the **femoral artery**. The radiologist watches on a TV screen while he or she inserts a long, thin tube called a catheter into the artery and pushes it along carefully until it reaches the point where the artery branches into several smaller vessels that feed the uterus (see Figure 7–1).

Once the catheter is in place, tiny plastic grains made of polyvinyl alcohol (PVA) or gelatin sponge are released, clogging the vessels that feed the uterus. The procedure is then repeated for the opposite side.

The whole procedure takes about 1 hour, after which you will be observed for another hour or two for pain symptoms. During

Figure 7–1. Fibroid Embolization

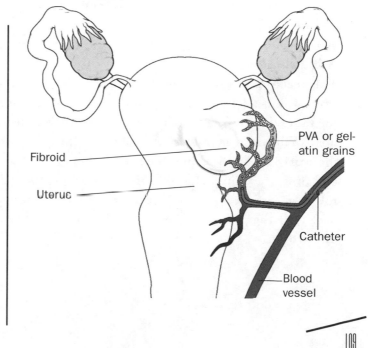

This technique starves fibroids of their blood supply by clogging the uterine arteries with tiny grains.

Fibroid

Uterus

PVA or gelatin grains

Catheter

Blood vessel

and immediately following embolization, you'll experience cramping that ranges from minimal to very painful in some patients. Most of the severe pain usually subsides after 12 hours and the remaining pain can be controlled with painkillers. You'll be given pain medication in the hospital and a prescription before going home. Pain may last for up to 2 weeks.

You may also experience a brownish discharge from your vagina and sometimes soft, jelly-like fibroids will be passed. A slight fever is common, but if your temperature rises above 38 degrees C (100 degrees F) you should contact your doctor. Most women return to normal daily activities within a week.

Advantages

This technique is very effective for heavy bleeding, which usually slows within 24 hours. In fact, uterine embolization has been used for more than two decades to stop uncontrolled bleeding after childbirth. Fibroids generally start to shrink within 6 weeks and are half their original size within 6 months. Other symptoms such as pain and pressure should also diminish. According to studies that have followed women for up to 6 years, fibroids do not appear to grow back after the procedure, except during pregnancy due to high levels of estrogen.

There were some worries that uterine embolization might ruin a woman's sex life, but they appear to be unfounded. Women with large fibroids often complain of painful intercourse and bloating affecting their sex life, so the procedure may actually improve sex for these women. Recent surveys show that some women report increased sexual desire and more intense orgasms after the procedure.

Disadvantages

A serious risk of uterine fibroid embolization is decreased fertility, due to reduced blood flow to the ovaries. It also appears to trigger early menopause in 1 in 100 women. Although pregnancy is possible following embolization, there appears to be a higher risk of miscarriage or premature birth, so if you plan to get pregnant, it is not your best choice. Another downside is the risk of a severe infection of the uterus, but this is rare.

"For my embolization I didn't know what to expect. At first I thought, 'this isn't too bad' and then they started on the third fibroid and it was agony. I don't know what they gave me, but it made me feel really sick and didn't make the pain go away. Once I got home all I did was sleep for 5 days. I couldn't even eat. They did tell me I would be in pain until the fibroids shrank, but I didn't realize how much pain. I found out later that the hospital now does an epidural right away."

Susan

Endometrial Ablation

What Is It?

Endometrial ablation, which was first performed in 1979, is a more sophisticated and effective version of a D&C. Used to treat excessive uterine bleeding without a hysterectomy, it involves inserting a device through the vagina into the uterus to destroy the uterine lining. Endometrial ablation is performed under a general, regional, or local anesthetic.

Depending on what kind of technique your physician will use, you may need to take a drug such as Lupron (see page 107) for 4 weeks before the procedure to thin out the lining of the uterus and shrink your fibroids. You generally go home the same day as your procedure and resume normal activities within 1 to 2 weeks, although you may continue to have vaginal discharge for up to 8 weeks.

There are many kinds of endometrial ablation devices, using electricity, heat, laser or microwave energy, or freezing. Endometrial ablation can be performed with or without hysteroscopy, in which the surgeon uses a small camera to see inside the uterus while he or she is performing the procedure.

Your physician should always rule out other causes of excessive bleeding before recommending uterine ablation, especially non-hysteroscopic ablation where he or she will not be able to see inside the uterus. Polyps, fibroids, or even uterine cancer may be missed during non-hysteroscopic endometrial ablation. Endometrial biopsy beforehand is a must in order to rule out cancer.

Some physicians combine endometrial ablation with fibroid removal by hysteroscopy. This can work well for fibroids located inside the uterine cavity (submucous fibroids). However, fibroids in the wall of the uterus (intramural fibroids) cannot be seen or removed by hysteroscopy, so if you have this kind of fibroid, the combination approach is not available to you.

Hysteroscopic Devices

There are several types of hysteroscopic endometrial ablation devices. These devices are inserted into the uterus through a channel along the side of the hysteroscope so the physician can see what he or she is doing at all times. The **roller ball technique** involves using a metal ball like a tiny steamroller to burn away the uterine lining in strips using electrosurgery (see Figure 7–2). In **loop endometrial ablation**, electricity is delivered to a tiny loop wire that is used to shave off the uterine lining and some of the deeper tissue, like mowing a lawn all the way to its roots. This is also called **endometrial resection**. A technique called **hydrothermal ablation**

Figure 7–2. Endometrial Ablation

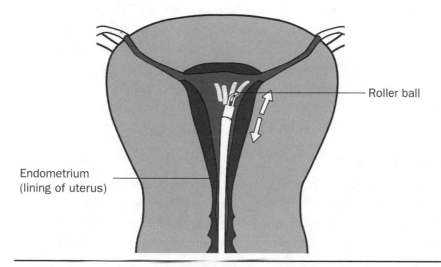

Roller ball

Endometrium
(lining of uterus)

This procedure destroys the lining of the uterus with an instrument inserted through the vagina. In this illustration, a roller ball uses an electrical current to destroy the tissue.

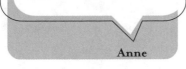

"They did a hysteroscopy to look inside the uterus and confirm what they found on ultrasound and then they did the endometrial ablation and then the resection of the fibroid. They do this at the same time as the ablation. They just work away at it, and take out as much as they can."

Anne

involves destroying the endometrium with a hot solution. The tissue turns from pink to white when the ablation is complete.

Non-Hysteroscopic Devices

In procedures where hysteroscopy is not used, the doctor inserts an instrument inside the uterus and destroys the uterine lining without seeing it. It is less demanding and easier to perform than hysteroscopic ablation. There are several different devices that appear to be equally effective. **Uterine balloon therapy devices** are inserted into the uterus via the cervix and then inflated. Some are filled with water that is then heated (e.g., Thermachoice or Cavaterm). Other devices use microwaves or laser energy to destroy the uterine lining. A **bipolar device** (Novasure) involves delivering electricity directly to the endometrium through a fan-like device that opens up after being placed in the uterus. **Cryoablation** uses cold instead of heat and freezes the uterine lining under ultrasound guidance.

Advantages

In the short-term, endometrial ablation has many advantages over hysterectomy. The procedure is faster and less invasive than hysterectomy and the recovery time is less—about 3 weeks, or half that of hysterectomy. About 20 percent of women have no bleeding 2 to 3 years after the operation, and 50 to 60 percent have reduced bleeding.

Alternatives to Hysterectomy— Essential Questions to Ask ✓

- ○ What will this treatment do for me?

- ○ What will happen if I don't have it?

- ○ What are the alternatives?

- ○ What are the pros and cons of this treatment compared to a hysterectomy?

- ○ What are the chances that it won't make any difference?

- ○ What are the chances that it will cure my symptoms?

- ○ Might it make me worse?

- ○ What are the risks?

- ○ How will it affect my sex life? My fertility?

- ○ How long will I take to recover afterward?

- ○ Would you recommend it if I was your partner/daughter/mother? (Go on—you can ask this one!)

- ○ How many times have you done this procedure before? (You can ask this one, too!)

Disadvantages

On the other hand, unlike hysterectomy, endometrial ablation does not guarantee to stop all bleeding in the future. One in five women finds no improvement (or the bleeding gets worse) and they need a repeat ablation or a hysterectomy. If you are hoping that endometrial ablation will stop your periods permanently, you are likely to be disappointed. Endometrial ablation also affects fertility, so it is not the best choice for women who still want children. It's also unsuitable for women with large fibroids or cancer. Generally, the results are better in women over age 40 than in younger women.

Although complications following endometrial ablation are less common than after hysterectomy, they still happen in 2 to 6 percent of women. Infection, problems with the anesthetic, and excessive bleeding are risks, as with any surgery. Absorption of fluids used to flush out the uterus in some techniques can lead to fluid overload and put a strain on the heart. Rarely, an ablation instrument may pierce the wall of the uterus, which would need to be repaired with surgery.

Myomectomy

What Is It?

Myomectomy is a procedure usually performed under a general anesthetic in which only the fibroids (or myomas) are scooped out, leaving the uterus intact (see Figure 7–3). It is designed for women who still want children or simply don't want a hysterectomy. Traditionally, it is done through the abdominal wall (**abdominal myomectomy**). Increasingly, it is also done through the vagina by hysteroscopy or by laparoscopy, depending on whether the fibroids are inside or outside the uterus.

Hysteroscopic myomectomy is for fibroids on the inside of the uterus and is the least invasive technique because the surgeon enters the uterus through the natural passage of the vagina. He or she uses a hysteroscope (Figure 2–2 on page 41), a long telescope that is inserted into the uterus to allow the surgeon to see into the uterus during the procedure, which is done on an outpatient basis and takes about 30 minutes. Recovery after hysteroscopic myomectomy is faster, with fewer complications, compared to laparoscopic or abdominal myomectomy. It may not be possible for women with severe bleeding problems or large fibroids.

Laparoscopic myomectomy takes 1 to 2 hours and may not require an overnight stay in the hospital. It involves 3 or 4 small incisions in the abdomen, but recovery is usually faster than in

Figure 7–3. Myomectomy

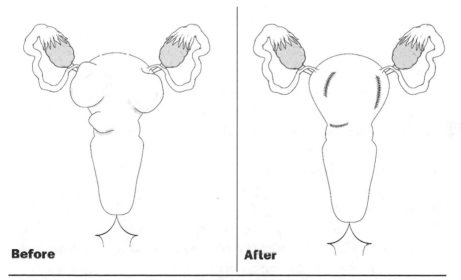

Before   **After**

Myomectomy is the surgical removal of fibroids from the uterus. It can be performed through an abdominal incision or by using a laparoscope. If the fibroids project into the uterus, a hysteroscope (a surgical telescope through the vagina) can be used instead.

abdominal myomectomy. It is used for fibroids on the outside of the uterus or inside the uterine wall. Again, it may not be possible for women with very large fibroids.

Abdominal myomectomy involves an 8 cm (3 inch) cut in the abdomen, either vertical from the belly button downward or a horizontal "bikini cut" above your pubic hair. This approach is needed for very large or very numerous fibroids.

The procedure itself, which takes place under general anesthetic, is similar to shelling a boiled egg. The surgeon makes an incision in the wall of the uterus over the fibroid. The fibroid is then shelled out using either a laser or conventional surgical tools, and the opening on the uterus is stitched up.

Recovery from myomectomy depends on how it was done. You should be able to return to normal activities within a few days after hysteroscopic myomectomy, about 2 weeks after laparoscopic myomectomy, and about 6 weeks after abdominal myomectomy.

If you are hoping to conceive, you should wait at least 2 months before having unprotected sex to allow the uterus time to heal fully.

Advantages

The major advantage of myomectomy over hysterectomy is that your uterus and ovaries are left intact, and there is still the possibility of getting pregnant. Studies show that about 50 percent of women who want to conceive after myomectomy manage to do so (compared to zero percent for hysterectomy).

Disadvantages

On the other hand, myomectomy cannot guarantee that you will become pregnant if you want to, you may grow additional fibroids over time, and it may not cure your heavy bleeding. For these reasons myomectomy is not the obvious alternative to hysterectomy that it may seem to be at first. Also, myomectomy is a more technically challenging operation than hysterectomy and you are more at risk of complications (unwanted medical events), such as heavy bleeding. In rare cases, bleeding during the surgery may become so heavy that the surgeon will need to go ahead and do a hysterectomy after all; you may be asked to sign a consent form beforehand allowing the surgeon to do this. Not all surgeons are comfortable with myomectomy, and in this procedure, experience counts. Don't be afraid to ask your surgeon how many times he or she has done myomectomy before deciding whether to proceed with him or her.

Myolysis

What Is It?

Myolysis is a technique for shrinking fibroids in which the surgeon makes deep incisions in the fibroid using a laser or long, heated needles. This "kills" the fibroid by damaging the small blood vessels that feed it with blood and it gradually shrinks. An experimental technique called **cryomyolysis**, in which the tissue is frozen for several minutes instead of heated, is also in development. Myolysis is carried out under laparoscopy (Figure 6–3), so it involves a general anesthetic, a day in hospital, and 3 or 4 small incisions in your abdomen. Recovery takes 1 to 2 weeks.

Advantages

The main advantage of myolysis is that your uterus is preserved and you avoid the risks of an abdominal surgical procedure such as myomectomy.

Disadvantages

The downside is that myolysis can cause **adhesions** (scar tissue) that can cause infertility, abdominal pain, and, possibly, intestinal obstruction. There is also a slight risk that your uterus will rupture during a future pregnancy. It is therefore not recommended for women who want to have a baby. It is better to remove the fibroids altogether, if needed.

Treatments for Cervical Dysplasia

What Are They?

Cervical dysplasia or "precancer" of the cervix (see page 26) can clear up by itself, so your physician may recommend a watch and wait approach for a while, including more regular Pap tests.

If treatment is needed, there are several options, but the basic idea is to remove the suspicious-looking tissue. Surgical treatments include laser surgery and cryosurgery, which freezes the tissue with nitrogen gas. These two surgical approaches are gradually being replaced by a third option, loop electrosurgical excision procedure or LEEP. This relatively new technique involves slicing off the suspicious cells with a thin, electrified wire loop. The cells can then be sent for testing, so LEEP doubles as a diagnostic procedure. If cancer cells are found, further treatment will be planned.

All these procedures can be done in your doctor's office under local anesthetic. You may have a little bleeding and cramping for a few hours after laser surgery or cryosurgery.

A **cone biopsy** involves removing a cone-shaped sample of tissue from around the opening of the cervix. It is done under a general anesthetic and you will need to be admitted to hospital for the day. It is both a diagnostic procedure (because the cells are sent away for laboratory testing) and a treatment (because it may remove all the suspicious tissue).

Advantages and Disadvantages

The advantage of all these treatments is that they are very successful at preventing cervical dysplasia from progressing to cancer. LEEP involves much less discomfort than all the other surgical options, with few short- or long-term problems. The downside of all the surgical procedures is that they can weaken the cervix, making future pregnancies a little more tricky.

Options for Uterine Prolapse

What Are They?

Although hysterectomy tends to be the treatment of choice if your prolapse is severe, it is by no means the only option. Exercises to strengthen the pelvic floor may help if your prolapse is mild (see Kegel exercises, page 168). If you are post-menopausal, your physician may prescribe an estrogen cream that you apply to your vagina to thicken the supporting tissues. Premenopausal women with severe prolapse who still want children may benefit from reconstructive surgery (AP repair, page 97). A useful interim measure if you have a severe prolapse but want more children, or are not well enough to undergo surgery right away, is a device called a **pessary** that is inserted into your vagina by your physician.

Advantages and Disadvantages

The advantage of all the above treatments is that they preserve your uterus, perhaps long enough for you to have children. However, if you have a severe prolapse, all the alternatives have serious disadvantages that may make hysterectomy inevitable in the end. Estrogen creams and exercises are ineffective for severe prolapse. Pessaries are just an interim measure and can cause chafing, discomfort, and infection. Reconstructive surgery is a major procedure with all the attendant risks and discomfort.

What Happens Next?

If you decide to go through with a procedure, the next stage is to recover your energy and health, and move on positively with your life. The next chapter discusses recovery from hysterectomy, but many of the suggestions are also helpful for getting over any major procedure.

Chapter 8

when it's all over

What Happens in this Chapter

- The recovery room
- Your return to the ward
- Pain management
- Care of your wound
- Eating, drinking, and going to the bathroom
- Going home checklist

After your hysterectomy, you will spend several hours in the recovery room. You will need to stay in bed until you are fully awake. After being transferred to the ward, your friends and family will be able to visit you and the nursing staff will keep an eye on you to check that all is well. You will then be allowed to go home.

The Recovery Room

As soon as your hysterectomy is over, you will be transferred—still lying flat—to the recovery room. You will be observed for about 2 hours until you wake up from the anesthesia. When you wake up, you will be groggy and have a small tube in your nose or a clear mask that is feeding you oxygen. Although you will probably feel relieved that your surgery is over, you may start to feel discomfort. Don't hesitate to ask the nursing staff for pain medication. It is also not unusual to feel nauseous and throw up after surgery due to the anesthetic. Your nurse can give you medication to help with this. If you know you've had trouble with nausea in the past, tell your doctor and anesthesiologist ahead of time. They can give you medication to prevent nausea.

> "I had 3 little cuts and they went in through my bellybutton. It was wonderful. The doctor was there for me, and he reassured my boyfriend that everything was going to be fine."
>
> **Betty**

Bleeding Is Normal   [MORE DETAIL]

It is normal to see a small amount of blood from your incisions through your bandages. If the nursing staff feels that the bleeding is excessive, they will call your doctor, or his or her assistant, to look at your wounds. Usually, an additional pressure bandage is all that is needed to stop the bleeding. You should also expect light bleeding from your vagina.

Arrival Back on the Ward

After your hysterectomy, your medical team will do everything to make sure that you have a safe recovery. In order to prevent problems from arising, and to ensure that complications are dealt with quickly, the following sequence of events will occur:

- The nurse accompanying you from the recovery room will give a short report to the ward nurse. This will include information about your hysterectomy, a brief summary of your condition in the recovery room, the medication you were given, special care instructions, and any other information related to your recovery process.

- The ward nurse will take your pulse, blood pressure, and temperature frequently until your condition is stable.

- Your bandages will be checked regularly for signs of bleeding.

- The nurse will make sure you don't have excessive vaginal bleeding.

- Your intravenous line will be checked regularly to ensure that it is working properly and that the correct doses of medication and fluids are being delivered to you. The nurse will refill the intravenous bag when it is almost empty.

- The nurse will carry out the physician's written orders, including the amount and frequency of medication.

Post-Hysterectomy Pain

It is normal for you to experience pain after your hysterectomy. Immediately after your surgery, you will receive pain medication every 3 to 4 hours. It is important to take pain medication on a regular basis because it's easier to prevent pain than it is to try to get it under control once it has worsened. Once your pain is consistently under control, your painkillers can be reduced.

Controlling your pain is an important part of your recovery because the less pain you're in, the better you will recover.

Don't rely on your physician and the nursing staff to guess when and how much you are in pain. You should play an active role in your pain control by letting your medical team know how they can make you more comfortable.

Get a Grip on Pain

[MORE DETAIL]

Poorly controlled pain can lead to complications. The more effective your pain control, the faster your recovery. Don't hesitate to tell your medical team if you are in pain.

Good Pain Control Means	Why Is This Important?
Being able to breathe and cough easily	It lowers your risk of pneumonia
Being able to walk easily	It helps prevent blood clots
Being able to sleep well	It helps you heal faster

Types of Pain Medication

There are two types of pain medications: **narcotics** and **non-narcotics**. The most common narcotics used after a hysterectomy are morphine or Demerol, and tablets consisting of codeine and its derivatives. You are usually given a stool softener along with your medication because narcotics can make you constipated.

Examples of non-narcotic medications include ASA (e.g., Aspirin), acetaminophen (e.g., Tylenol), ibuprofen (e.g., Advil), and naproxen (e.g., Anaprox). These medications are in pill form and will only be given to you after you are able to drink. You may also be given a potent non-narcotic through your I.V. line called ketorolac (e.g., Toradol).

[**KEY POINT**]

Some patients worry about taking narcotics, such as morphine and codeine, because they are afraid that they will become addicted to them. However, it is rare to become dependent on narcotics when you are using them to control pain. People who become addicted to narcotics usually already have some form of substance-abuse problem.

Pain Control with the Touch of a Button

One extremely effective way to control pain following an abdominal hysterectomy, is with a **patient-controlled analgesia (PCA)** pump. With PCA, a pump filled with pain medication (usually morphine) is connected directly to your intravenous or epidural line. By pressing a button on this pump, you can give yourself an amount of medication specified by your doctor.

The PCA pump has a safety timer called a **lock-out**, so you won't overdose yourself. If you press the pump button during the lock-out time, you won't receive medicine because there is a limit to the amount of pain medication you can safely receive within any 4 hours.

Once you press the button, the pain medicine should take 5 to 10 minutes to work. The PCA pump is usually removed the day after your hysterectomy and you will then be given narcotics via injections in your buttock muscle to control your pain or strong pills once you are tolerating food without nausea. Here is a list of do's and don'ts for your PCA pump:

DO...

- press the button when you start to feel pain
- use the pump before you move or turn, do breathing and coughing exercises, or anything else that is likely to be painful

DO NOT...

- wait until your pain is bad before using the pump
- let others press the button on your pump
- use the PCA for gas pain
- press the button when you are comfortable and sleepy.

Intravenous PCA

If your PCA pump is connected to your intravenous line, you may experience certain side effects. You might feel sleepy or nauseous, and you may vomit. Your skin may also itch and you might find it hard to urinate. If you experience any of these side effects mention them to your nurse.

Epidural PCA

If you had an epidural during your hysterectomy (see page 93), your medical team may decide that maintaining your epidural for up to 2 days would be helpful in controlling your pain. If your epidural is left in place, your PCA pump may be attached to it.

Your epidural will make your legs heavy and numb and it will be hard for you to move around. Your nurse will check regularly to see if your lack of mobility becomes a problem. You may also experience specific side effects from your PCA epidural, such as nausea, vomiting, dizziness, sleepiness, difficulty urinating, and itchy skin. Your nurse can give you pain medication if you develop a headache or backache from your epidural PCA. Some rare complications of an epidural include transient numbness, weakness, or paralysis, and allergic reactions, seizures, or a heart attack.

Local Anesthesia Pain Pump

Some centers may offer you a new option called a **local anesthesia pain pump**. This miniature "soaker hose" delivers local anesthesic directly to your incisions continually for about 3 days. Because it is portable, the pain pump makes it easy for you to move around while you recover.

The First Few Days After Your Hysterectomy

You may stay in the hospital for the first few days of your recovery so that your medical team can make sure that you are healing properly and as comfortably as possible. Your gynecologic surgeon, or his or her assistant, will check on you every day, so don't be afraid to ask any questions or raise concerns that you might have about your recovery.

Your Intravenous Line

For a while after your hysterectomy, you will receive fluid intravenously. Once you are able to drink normally and your bowel function has started to return to normal, your nurse will remove your intravenous line. The amount of time it takes before your intravenous line is removed varies from procedure to procedure. The intravenous line can usually be removed within 24 hours after laparoscopic and vaginal hysterectomies; however, it may take another day for the line to be removed after an abdominal hysterectomy.

Breathing and Coughing

One of the most important therapies for your recovery, particularly after an abdominal hysterectomy, is coughing. This might seem strange because your surgery had nothing to do with your lungs. However, mucus accumulates in your lungs during and immediately after any surgery. Coughing dislodges this mucus and helps prevent pneumonia. Coughing exercises need to be done frequently, about every 15 minutes. The exercise is simple: you sit up, take a deep breath, and cough strongly while pressing your abdomen with a pillow to reduce the pain. Spit out any mucus that you cough up into a tissue. You will also have to do breathing exercises to re-expand your lungs. To complete these exercises you may use a device called an **incentive spirometer**, which gives you feedback on how deep your breaths are.

"When I came home, I had to call my doctor because I kept having a very high temperature and I was so sick I thought I had pneumonia. So he gave me extra antibiotics. My belly also felt a little swollen and I was always having difficulty urinating."

Silvia

Temperature and Vital Signs

Your nurses will keep careful track of your temperature and vital signs (pulse and blood pressure) to make sure that there are no signs of infection or other complications. Each time a new nurse starts a shift, he or she will check how you are doing. There are usually three nursing shifts in a 24-hour rotation: morning, afternoon, and night. Therefore, you will probably be checked at least three times a day.

Bladder Function

If your hysterectomy was uncomplicated and a bladder catheter was left in, your nurse will probably remove your catheter the day after your surgery. However, if your bladder was repaired or a urethral suspension (see page 97) was done during your hysterectomy, your catheter will be left in longer. It may take about 8 hours for you to urinate after your catheter is removed. Once your catheter is out, a nurse or a family member can help you go to the bathroom. At night, feel free to ask the nurse for a bedpan so that you don't have to walk all the way to the bathroom.

Don't worry if you feel discomfort the first few times that you urinate after surgery—this is not unusual. If you continue to feel pain while urinating, you should inform your nurse or a member of your medical team because you may have a bladder infection. If you cannot urinate, or just a small amount of urine comes out even though your bladder is full, a catheter may be reinserted for an extra day.

> "My incisions didn't hurt unless I touched them and I had a little discomfort when I passed urine, just over the pubic bone, but basically I felt great."
>
> **Dawn**

Bowel Function

Asking someone whether she has passed gas is usually considered impolite. However, following a hysterectomy or any other abdominal operation, you will be asked this question on many occasions. The manipulation of your intestines during your hysterectomy, especially if your surgeon went the abdominal route, will make your intestines sluggish, so tracking when you pass gas is one way to know whether or not your bowel function is back to normal. The doctor will also listen to your abdomen with a stethoscope for bowel sounds.

Once you have passed gas or have bowel sounds, you will be allowed to drink and will eventually have a bowel movement.

Help Yourself to Less Bloating

It's normal to experience bloating and gas cramps when your first start drinking. There are several ways to make this painful gas pass quickly. Walking, or drinking warm water, prune juice, or tea can be helpful. Your physician may also give you laxatives, such as glycerin suppositories or milk of magnesia, or offer you chewable tablets containing simethicone.

However, having your first bowel movement after surgery may take some time. You may be constipated because you will not have eaten solid food for a day or two. Pain medications such as morphine and codeine will also contribute to your constipation. You may not even have a bowel movement by the time you are discharged.

Eating and Drinking

Many patients do not have a large appetite after surgery. You may feel nauseous due to the anesthesia or narcotics and your pain medication will decrease your appetite. In fact, you may not be hungry at all. If you are feeling nauseous, inform your nurse or physician. There are medications that can help relieve your nausea.

Most patients can tolerate a fluid diet the day of laparoscopic or vaginal hysterectomy, but it might take 2 to 3 days for patients who have had an abdominal hysterectomy to be able to tolerate it. Once you are able to eat a fluid diet, you can start eating regular food.

Vaginal Bleeding

Following a hysterectomy, it is normal to experience a small amount of vaginal bleeding, which might be slightly heavier than that of your normal menstrual flow. If the blood is excessive and smells bad, you should inform your nurse or another member of your medical team.

Your Incisions

Your incisions will be monitored carefully by the medical staff to make sure that there are no signs of infection or blood collecting under the skin (**hematoma**). Usually, your physician will remove your bandages on the third day after surgery. You can then take a shower and wash your wounds gently with soap. After bathing, you should dry your incisions thoroughly. If you aren't comfortable with leaving your incisions uncovered you can ask your nurse to apply a light dressing.

If your incisions are closed with staples or clips, they will be removed on the fourth or fifth day after your hysterectomy. If you are discharged early, you should make an appointment to have your staples or clips removed. Your physician, or his or her assistant, will sometimes apply thin transparent tapes called **Steri-strips** to keep the edges of the wound together. These tapes will eventually fall off after several weeks.

If you have had a vaginal hysterectomy, you won't have any abdominal incisions. However, if a long piece of gauze was inserted into your vagina immediately after your surgery (vaginal pack), it will be removed a day or two after your operation. The sutures to close your vaginal incision will simply dissolve and do not have to be removed.

Physical Activity

Moving around after surgery can be hard, but it is very important to your recovery and the nursing staff will provide you with lots of support the first few times you get out of bed. Your medical team wants you to be up and walking within a day of your operation to prevent blood clots from forming in your legs. Walking also stimulates movement in your intestines, so your digestion can return to normal more quickly and you can start eating normal food sooner.

However, while you are too groggy and weak to get up, you will be encouraged to move your legs while in bed and your nurse will help you turn from side to side. The first time you attempt to get up will be the toughest. Be aware that after experiencing anesthesia and lying in your hospital bed for several hours, you might feel dizzy and your legs may be weak when you try to stand. That's why a nurse will assist you the first time you attempt to get up. He or she will ask you to sit with your legs dangling down the side of the bed. Then your nurse will help you sit in a chair. This process will be repeated several times a day. If you begin to feel strong enough, you can even walk to the bathroom. If you still have an intravenous line, your nurse will give you an intravenous pole so that you can walk with it.

Blood Tests

Following an abdominal or vaginal hysterectomy, blood tests may be taken on the day after your surgery to make sure that you are not anemic. If your hemoglobin and blood-iron levels are low, you will be prescribed iron pills. If you have the actual symptoms of anemia, such as dizziness, fatigue, breathlessness, fainting, or lightheadedness, your physician may suggest a blood transfusion.

Friends and Family

[KEY POINT]

If you are too tired to have visitors, it is advisable to have only your immediate family or close friends stay with you. You can also ask the hospital operator to hold any telephone calls until you are feeling stronger.

After your hysterectomy, your friends and family will be anxious to see you. However, your safety must come first. Before you are allowed visitors, the nursing and medical staff will check that your condition is stable. Once you are stable, your family or friends will be allowed to see you.

Pre-Discharge Consultation

Before you are sent home, you will be seen by your physician, or his or her assistant, and by a nurse for your pre-discharge consultation. Now is the time to ask any questions, such as how successful your hysterectomy was, and what to do in the event of emergency. Once your questions have been answered, your physician or nurse will provide you with a great deal of information and advice. It's a good idea to have a friend or a family member present during your consultation to help you remember the information and, possibly, write it down. Your hospital may also provide you with an information sheet.

Leaving the Hospital

Use this hospital checklist to make sure you have everything you need for your recovery at home:

- A letter to your referring physician   ○
- A letter to your employer or insurance company   ○
- An appointment to have your staples or clips removed (if needed)   ○
- Prescriptions for painkillers and any other medications (if needed)   ○
- A contact name and number in case of an emergency   ○
- A general information package, including a list of do's and don'ts   ○
- Someone to escort you home   ○
- A follow-up appointment   ○
- Your personal items   ○
- This book!   ○

What Happens Next?

Once you are discharged and at home, your healing process will continue. Now it is up to you to get lots of rest and then gradually ease into your regular routine.

Chapter 9

recovering at home

What Happens in this Chapter

- Your first day at home
- Your medication
- Caring for your incisions
- Eating and going to the bathroom
- Vaginal bleeding and discharge
- What to do in an emergency
- Guidelines for getting back to work
- Exercise, driving and flying
- Your sex life
- Your emotions
- Follow-up visits

You're finally back at home and you can take the time you need to rest and fully heal. Although the first few days after your hysterectomy will not be easy, you are past the most difficult part of your recovery. By following a few simple guidelines and gradually increasing your activity, you will soon be back to your normal routine.

Your First Day at Home

Once you are back at home, it is important to rest so that you can heal properly. However, maintaining a certain activity level is an essential part of your recovery. The earlier you walk, the faster you will get better. Everyone is different, so listen to your body and do what feels best for you.

[S E L F - H E L P]

Recovery Do's and Don'ts

DO...

- Take it easy
- Get plenty of rest
- Eat a healthy diet, with plenty of fruits and vegetables and lots of water
- Return to walking and gentle movement
- Try self-help techniques, such as relaxation or massage
- Keep stress at a minimum
- Quit smoking

DON'T...

- Rush back to work
- Forget that your incisions need time to heal
- Take your narcotics if you don't need them
- Do any heavy lifting or strenuous exercise
- Forget to take your prescribed medications
- Allow yourself to get stressed
- Continue to smoke

Your Medications

After your hysterectomy you will probably need to take a few different kinds of medications: painkillers and (maybe) antibiotics and
hormone therapy. You may wish to keep track of your medicines
using the diary pages in the back of this book.

Because the painkillers you take may
have side effects, such as constipation,
only take them if you feel you need
them. However, don't hesitate to
take your pain medication if you are
uncomfortable. The first few days
after you return home, you may
need pain medication as frequently
as every 4 hours. Once you have
used all of your prescribed pain
pills, you can buy acetaminophen
(e.g., Tylenol) at the pharmacy without a prescription if you still
need pain relief. However, don't mix over-the-counter medicines
with prescription medicines unless your physician has said it's safe.

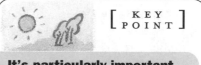

[KEY POINT]

It's particularly important
to be free of pain before
going to bed; getting a good
night's sleep will help you
recover faster.

Many women wonder whether they will need hormone replacement after their hysterectomy. If your ovaries have not been
removed, you will continue to produce estrogen and will not need to
take hormone pills. However, if both of your ovaries were removed
during your hysterectomy, your doctor will prescribe hormonal
replacement therapy (HRT) to treat menopausal symptoms such as
hot flushes, a dry vagina, and mood swings. Be aware that not all
women are candidates for HRT. For example, if you have
endometrial or breast cancer, you may not be eligible for HRT (see
Chapter 12).

Caring for Your Incisions

Before you leave the hospital, your physician, or his or her assistant, will check to make sure that your incisions are healing well. Once you're at home, it's easy to care for your wounds yourself. Treat them like any cut. Feel free to take showers, and wash your wounds gently with soap and dry them. If an incision is covered with Steri-strips, do not remove them. These strips will fall off by themselves after repeated showers, or you can pull them off when the ends of the strips curl. You should wait at least another 2 weeks before bathing in a bathtub. Your incisions do not have to be covered, but avoid wearing tight clothing that rubs against them.

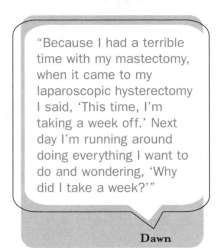

[**KEY POINT**]

Don't apply alcohol, hydrogen peroxide, or other solutions to your wounds because they may become irritated and heal more slowly.

It is common to see some bruising around your incisions. Your skin will look bluish and, after several days, will turn yellow before returning to its normal color. If you feel excessive pain near any of your incisions, especially if the area is red and swollen, contact your physician. You might have an infection and you may need antibiotics. Don't be alarmed if you have an infection—it is usually superficial and can be easily treated.

"Because I had a terrible time with my mastectomy, when it came to my laparoscopic hysterectomy I said, 'This time, I'm taking a week off.' Next day I'm running around doing everything I want to do and wondering, 'Why did I take a week?'"

Dawn

Physical Activity and Exercise

Although your incisions and abdomen may hurt, it's important that you increase your physical activity level. Start gradually by walking and don't overdo it. If you have stairs at home, you can go up and down slowly, one step at a time. Avoid pushing, lifting heavy objects, or doing strenuous activity for about 4 weeks after laparoscopic subtotal hysterectomy, and 6 weeks after total abdominal, laparoscopic or vaginal hysterectomy.

"When I had some bleeding after surgery, one of the doctors at the emergency was actually quite rude. She said, 'Well, after a laparoscopy, in a week people are up and running.' So I said, 'Well, as you can see, I'm not up and I'm not running either."

Silvia

[S E L F - H E L P]

Getting Things Moving

Even if your appetite is good, it is common to be constipated due to your pain medication. Try eating more raw fruits, vegetables, bran cereals, and whole-wheat breads to increase your fiber intake. Drinking prune juice and several glasses of water will also help to relieve your constipation. Talk to your physician if your constipation won't go away so that he or she can recommend a mild stool softener, such as Colace, or a laxative. If you have always had trouble with chronic constipation, don't wait! Begin with stool softeners, fiber supplements, and a mild laxative as soon as you get home.

Once your incisions have healed, you may gradually resume your regular exercise routine. However, it's best to wait for about 6 weeks after surgery before swimming, jogging, lifting weights, or doing any vigorous activity. Your body needs those calories to heal!

Eating and Going to the Bathroom

"At first my stomach was swollen—I looked 6 months pregnant. About 2 weeks after, my boyfriend took me to a restaurant and I had to wear a maternity outfit, loose pants and a top. We finished supper and he wanted the bill, so he tells the waitress to hurry up because my waters are about to break!"

Betty

Once you are home, you may eat normally. Don't worry if you aren't very hungry. Just eat small but more frequent portions and remember to drink plenty of fluids.

You may also have trouble urinating or have painful urination. The irritation caused by your bladder catheterization before and immediately after your hysterectomy may have caused a bladder infection. Be assured that most infections are not serious and can be cured with antibiotics. Drinking a lot of liquids after your hysterectomy will help prevent bladder irritation.

Vaginal Bleeding and Discharge

You will have a brownish-red vaginal discharge for 4 to 6 weeks after your hysterectomy. Don't be alarmed—this is normal. Your discharge could last even longer if you've had a subtotal hysterectomy, due to the process of sealing the cervix at the end of this procedure. It is important that you *do not* try vaginal douching to clean out your discharge. Douching removes normal bacteria that keep the vagina healthy. As you become more active during weeks 2-3, the amount of bleeding and discharge may actually increase. Don't be alarmed—this is normal as the stitches dissolve.

[**KEY POINT**]

Avoid using tampons for about 4 weeks after your surgery because they could irritate the vaginal incision and cause abnormal bleeding. Douching is also a bad idea because it encourages abnormal bacteria or fungi to grow in your vagina.

What to Do in an Emergency

Contact your doctor or go to the emergency room if you are experiencing:

- fever of over 38°C or 100.2°F
- frequent or painful urination
- inability to pass gas and persistent vomiting
- painful, red, swollen, or odorous discharge from your incision
- heavy vaginal bleeding (soaking a pad an hour) or odorous discharge
- sudden pain in your chest
- flank pain
- one-sided calf swelling and pain

Getting Back to Work

> "I was back to work after about 6 weeks. I had some leaking, and they thought my bladder was punctured, but I went for some tests and there was no problem, everything was fine. It just took time to heal on its own."
>
> **Betty**

After laparoscopic or vaginal surgery, you can return to part-time work within 2 weeks if you feel well. After abdominal hysterectomy, 6 weeks is a reasonable time. It is helpful to work half days your first week back (working the *second* half of the day to stop you working too many hours out of guilt). You can build your stamina gradually to return full-time.

Driving and Flying

> "I took a month off because when I got back I couldn't just go at half speed, and I also went into surgery tired and anemic—I wasn't feeling great. So you've got to get back to baseline first, and then you've got to recover."
>
> **Anne**

There is no law against driving after a hysterectomy. In general, you can start driving about 2 weeks after your surgery, but it also depends how much pain you're in and how strong you feel while you are recovering. If you are not experiencing abdominal pain and you feel strong enough to drive, you may start by driving around the block. If you experience sudden pain while driving, this is a sign that you are not ready. You should stop until the pain passes and return home immediately. You can then try driving again in 2 to 3 days. You should not drive if you still require pain medication, which could make you feel drowsy and make driving dangerous.

It is best to wait until at least 2 weeks after your operation before attempting to fly, even if you feel well enough before then.

Follow-Up Visits

Unless you experience an emergency (see page 143), your physician will advise you to make a follow-up appointment 2 to 6 weeks after your hysterectomy so that he or she can make sure that you have healed properly. At this visit, your doctor will examine your incisions and explain your pathology results. Hormone replacement therapy and lifestyle changes may also be discussed. A blood test is not usually needed, although your physician may want to check whether or not you are anemic.

Your Sex Life

The First Few Weeks

You probably won't feel much like having sex for the first couple of weeks after your surgery. You'll probably feel sore and tired and still have a vaginal discharge. However, people vary, so it's worth talking about the rules, and also defining what we mean by "sex."

When your physician or nurse advises you "not to have sex" for 4 to 6 weeks after your hysterectomy, he or she is talking about anything that involves inserting something into your vagina. You should wait at least 4 weeks after your hysterectomy before having sexual intercourse if your cervix is still in place. If you had a total hysterectomy, a wait of 6 weeks is safer. There is a very real worry that the vigorous friction of intercourse may burst your stitches. The 4- to 6-week rule also applies to anything that you might insert into your vagina, including fingers, a tampon, or even a douche, due to the risk of infection. So masturbation that involves inserting something into your vagina is inadvisable, too. Once you have healed, there may be some slight bleeding or staining the first few times you have intercourse. If this doesn't go away, or gets worse, contact your physician to be checked out.

So what about other types of "sex"? There is no evidence that orgasm itself will rupture stitches, so external genital stimulation to orgasm, either by your partner or yourself, is likely to be safe. Again, you may not feel very sexy as you recover, but if you do, go ahead and do what feels good as long as it doesn't involve actual intercourse. You can have fun experimenting with alternate ways to achieve orgasm for a while.

Don't forget, too, that the "no sex" rule doesn't apply to hugging, kissing, romantic dinners, or a mutual massage. If you are lucky enough to live with someone who cares about you, enjoy them and their loving touch just as much as you always did, and it might speed your healing.

The Long-Term Picture

"There was no change in my sex life afterwards. It depends on why you're having the surgery. I had it because I couldn't stand it anymore, so I was willing to deal with what I got. And I made the right decision—it's freedom, 24/7."

Anne

As we discussed in Chapter 1, your uterus does not have a big role to play in sexual satisfaction, so there is no reason to believe that after a hysterectomy your levels of satisfaction will be lower. Women who have had the cervix removed may be more likely to report a difference in their orgasms, but this is extremely rare, in our experience. Scar tissue may also create problems for some women. However, it may help to remember that the clitoris is the kingpin when it comes to sexual pleasure. All orgasms probably originate in the clitoris, whether an orgasm is felt as "vaginal" or "clitoral." This is why many women do not notice a difference in their orgasms after hysterectomy.

What Science Tells Us

So is it just a myth that hysterectomy ruins sex? What we do know is that, although there is a huge amount of individual variation, the problem is vastly over-exaggerated. One of the largest and most reliable studies, the Maryland Women's Health Study published in the prestigious *Journal of the American Medical Association* in 1999, found that sexual function actually improved overall after hysterectomy (see More Detail box on page 148). The group of women studied generally had more sex after hysterectomy and were able to reach orgasm more frequently.

But what about quality? Some women describe their orgasms as less intense after surgery. There could be many explanations for this. Although it is possible that surgery may have bruised, damaged, or removed nerves involved in your orgasm, you also have to consider factors that you can do something about—vaginal dryness, fatigue, or anxiety about your ability to "perform."

The Maryland Women's Health Study found that psychology was a powerful factor when it came to sexual problems after the surgery— women who were depressed before the procedure were the ones most likely to experience vaginal dryness, low libido, and lack of

[**KEY POINT**]

Remember, the brain is the most powerful sex organ of all. The belief that sex will be ruined by hysterectomy often becomes a self-fulfilling prophecy. Stay positive, stay imaginative, and go for it. There is rarely a good anatomical reason why sex shouldn't be just as fulfilling and enjoyable after surgery as beforehand, and if you encounter problems, there are plenty of solutions on hand.

"My sex life wasn't pleasant at the beginning, but now it's fine. I went off the hormone pills because of all the controversy, but I felt I was drying up and I didn't feel good; now I'm back on them and I feel better."

Betty

[**MORE DETAIL**]

The Maryland Women's Health Study, a good-quality study by researchers from the University of Maryland, found that, contrary to popular belief, sexual functioning actually *improved* after hysterectomy. The 2–year study tracked 1,100 women aged 35 to 49 before, and at 6, 12, 18, and 24 months after, hysterectomy. The results are shown below. The improvements could have been due to a number of factors, including freedom from bleeding and/or discomfort, or fear of pregnancy.

	Before Hysterectomy	2 Years After Hysterectomy
Never have sex	29%	23%
Sex frequently uncomfortable	19%	4%
Vaginal dryness	63%	54%
Cannot have an orgasm	8%	5%
Low libido	10%	6%

orgasms after hysterectomy. This is not really surprising, in view of the fact that, as we discussed in Chapter 1, the brain is the most powerful sex organ of all. A whole host of reasons may make some women feel less sexy after surgery, such as a different self-image, feeling unwell, a partner's attitude, or a perception that her "femininity" has gone. The belief that hysterectomy (or removal of the cervix) ruins sex may, of itself, be self-fulfilling: "I know it's not going to work." Be assured that there is rarely a good reason why you should not have just as good a sex life after hysterectomy as before—if not better.

Having said that, if you feel that your sex life is not as it should be, don't feel guilty or embarrassed. This is a complex area and everyone is different. If you feel comfortable with your physician, talk to him or her about it, and he or she should be able to refer you for tests or sex therapy. If you don't get the answers you need, change doctors. Chapter 10 offers some self-help advice you may wish to try.

The Role of Hormones

Hormones also have a part to play in sex after hysterectomy. If natural menopause is approaching, or you had your ovaries removed during your hysterectomy, you will have less estrogen in your body. Although estrogen does not affect sexual desire directly, the lack of estrogen will make your vagina and vulva drier and less flexible, so intercourse may be more uncomfortable (not surprisingly, this may reduce your interest in it). Also, less blood will flow to the vagina, clitoris, and breasts during arousal so they may feel less responsive, and orgasm may be more difficult to reach. Estrogen replacement therapy (see Chapter 12) will help with many of these symptoms. If you don't want to take artificial estrogen, there are many other things you can do to improve your sexual enjoyment (see page 166).

The hormone testosterone, which your ovaries produce in small amounts and has a role in your libido, also falls after

> "For the couple of months after surgery I felt strange, kind of empty and I was very vulnerable. I would get upset over any little thing, especially when I went back to the doctor and saw all those posters of the babies. I was jealous and upset that other women could have them and I couldn't anymore. I had no more chance."
>
> **Silvia**

menopause or surgical removal of your ovaries. Artificial testosterone can, therefore, help with sexual problems after hysterectomy
in some women.

Your Emotions

> "Afterwards you're emotionally a little bit like this and like that, but I know some women lose their uterus and it's the end of the world. I couldn't wait. It was the best thing that ever happened."
>
> Anne

The First Few Weeks

After the initial relief that it's all over, it's not uncommon to feel tired, weepy, emotional, and irritable after surgery. One day you're high, the next you've never felt lower. You're not sleeping properly, you're in pain, and no one can do anything right. However, be assured that as you start to heal and return to your normal activities you will start to feel better.

The Long-Term Picture

Many people believe that hysterectomy causes psychiatric problems such as depression and anxiety. This is a myth, based on old, poorly designed scientific studies. In fact, although there may be a short "mourning" period, there is no good evidence that hysterectomy causes long-term emotional problems if it is carried out for valid medical reasons. Studies also show that, generally speaking, women who do suffer emotional illness after hysterectomy are those who had problems before surgery.

If your recovery is painful and difficult, a lack of sleep, stress, and other factors common to all surgeries may also have a long-term effect on your emotional health. If you find that you really cannot pull yourself out of your black mood, see your physician, who will explore ways to help you.

If your ovaries have been removed (oophorectomy), you will suddenly enter menopause and experience menopausal symptoms such as hot flashes and vaginal dryness. Many women also suffer from depression or anxiety at this time and these "mood swings" are often blamed on lack of estrogen. In fact, the evidence that mood is related to hormone levels is shaky, and this belief owes more to the popular media than science. For many years scientists trying to unravel the puzzle of **premenstrual syndrome (PMS)** have tried to relate women's moods to estrogen levels in the blood and could not find a direct link. Some women find that estrogen replacement therapy helps with mood swings, others don't.

The bottom line is, "the blues" of menopause probably have less to do with estrogen and more to do with the fear of aging, interrupted sleep due to night sweats, and the humiliating and embarrassing onslaught of hot flashes. Estrogen replacement therapy appears to magically "improve mood" because it clears up these problems, allowing you to cope with life better.

What Happens Next?

Once you have recovered from your hysterectomy, you should be pain-free and your vaginal bleeding should have stopped. Remember, you still need a physical examination every year. Chapter 10 will give you tips on how to continue to care for yourself in the coming months.

Chapter

10

how you can help yourself

What Happens in this Chapter

- Healing after hysterectomy
- The impact of menopause
- Lifestyle shifts that can change your future
- Relaxation and complementary therapies
- Vitamins and herbs
- Improving your sex life
- Breast exams and Kegels

Any major medical procedure is a turning point in our lives. Life is never quite the same afterward—and it shouldn't be. Not only is it a reminder that life is precious, but it often brings into focus the things that we care about—and who cares for us. Friends, family, healthcare professionals, have lavished the best of themselves (and their training) on you and now it's your turn. Lavish care on yourself because you have a new life to live and you deserve the best. If you want to know how to love your bones, your heart, your mental health, or your sex life, both before and after menopause, this chapter will show you how.

Healing After Hysterectomy

HYSTERECTOMY IS A RELIEF FOR MANY WOMEN, RELEASING THEM from years of discomfort and inconvenience. As we discussed in Chapter 3, 8 out of 10 women said their health improved after hysterectomy. On the other hand, hysterectomy is a major procedure, so there is a recovery period like there is after any surgery. In addition, some women need time to come to terms with the fact that they no longer have a uterus and what this means for them personally. If you had your ovaries removed you will also be coping with the symptoms of menopause.

Healthy living can go a long way to helping with all these transitions. A good diet, plenty of exercise and sleep, no smoking, and regularly doing something that you enjoy add up to a simple but effective recipe for getting the best out of this new phase of your life. Complementary therapies, including herbal remedies, can also be powerful allies. There are also specific things you should be doing to ensure your long-term health after menopause and these are described below.

Managing Surgical Menopause

As we discussed in detail in Chapter 1, removal of your ovaries before the age of natural menopause causes a sudden decrease in the female hormones estrogen and progesterone and the male hormone testosterone. The sudden drop in estrogen will cause short-term problems such as hot flashes and night sweats (see page 17), and increase your long-term risk of osteoporosis, heart disease, and thinning of the vaginal wall (**atrophic vaginitis**). The decrease in blood testosterone may reduce your energy levels or sexual desire (see page 12).

Because of this, you will be offered hormone replacement therapy (HRT) to replace the hormones that are lacking (see Chapter 12). Herbal alternatives are also available. In addition, a healthy lifestyle is important. This includes a good diet that is rich in calcium, regular exercise, weight control, no smoking, and reduced caffeine and alcohol.

Take a Look at Your Diet

Calcium

Calcium has always been important, to keep your bones strong, but after menopause it is literally lifesaving. Osteoporosis, a condition in which your bones gradually become brittle and porous, becomes a very real possibility now that your estrogen levels have fallen. Eighty percent of hip fractures are due to osteoporosis and approximately 1 in 5 women die as a result. Eat more calcium!

Calcium is found in milk and other dairy products, fortified orange juice, dark leafy vegetables, and a host of other foods (see More Detail box). However, calcium in the diet alone is not enough. You need approximately 1,000 mg of elemental calcium daily combined with estrogen or 1,500 mg of elemental calcium daily without hormones. There are many calcium preparations and the amount of calcium in each is written on the package as "elemental calcium." The cheapest, yet the most rich with elemental calcium, is

calcium carbonate (40 percent). **Calcium citrate** is more easily absorbed than calcium carbonate, but it contains less elemental calcium (21 percent). Other preparations such as **calcium lactate** and **calcium gluconate** only contain 13 percent and 9 percent of elemental calcium respectively. Calcium is best taken with meals. Your body can only absorb about 500 mg of calcium at a time, so be sure that you are dividing your supplements into 2 or 3 servings. Side effects include constipation and (rarely) kidney stones. A calcium and magnesium combination will help you to avoid constipation.

Where Do I Find Calcium? [MORE DETAIL]

Food	How Much Calcium?
Skim milk, 1 cup	302 mg
Cheddar cheese, 1 oz/25 g	204 mg
Frozen yogurt, 1 cup/250 mL	240 mg
Ice cream, 1 cup/250 mL	176 mg
Canned salmon with bones, 3½ oz/100 g	185 mg
Cooked rhubarb, ½ cup/125 mL	174 mg
Cooked spinach, ½ cup/125 mL	138 mg
Tofu, ½ cup/125 mL	130 mg
Almonds, ¼ cup/50 mL	92 mg
Calcium carbonate tablets	
Calcite-500, Calcium 500, Os-Cal, Calcium Oyster Shell 500	500 mg
Calcite D-500, Calcium D 500, Os-Cal D, Calcium Oyster Shell 500 with vitamin D	500 mg and 125 IU vitamin D
Caltrate 600	600 mg
Caltrate 600+D	600 mg and 125 IU vitamin D
Caltrate Plus	600 mg, and 200 IU vitamin D, magnesium, zinc, copper, manganese

Vitamin D

Vitamin D is also essential for preventing osteoporosis. Your body produces this vitamin naturally when your skin is exposed to sunlight (it needs about 30 minutes a day), but obviously this can be a challenge in the northern United States. Vitamin D tablets are easily available, often combined with calcium. The recommended dose is 400 IU daily. After removal of your ovaries, you need about 1,000 mg of calcium and 400 IU of vitamin D daily. If you are not taking estrogen replacement therapy, you need 1,500 mg of calcium and 800 IU of vitamin D daily.

A Heart-Healthy Diet

Before menopause, women have lower rates of cardiovascular disease (heart attacks and strokes) than men. After natural or surgical menopause, they lose the protection of estrogen and their rates of cardiovascular disease start to climb, so a heart-healthy lifestyle becomes even more important than before. A heart-healthy diet involves eating a well-balanced diet high in fruit, vegetables, and fiber and low in saturated fats. Fresh fruit and lightly cooked vegetables will help to fill you up at meals so you will eat less high-fat food. They also contain active ingredients that fight disease, including heart disease.

Fiber will come along for the ride if you eat lots of fruit and vegetables and you can also find it in whole grains, nuts, and cereals (oatmeal, etc.).

Reducing fat in your diet often seems easier said than done. There are lots of confusing claims about heart-healthy fats, so it's best to keep the rules simple. Try to reduce your fat intake overall (by loading up your plate with fruit, vegetables, and fiber instead) and especially reduce **saturated fats**—the animal fats found in all those hamburgers and hot dogs.

Exercise

Exercise is important for all kinds of reasons after your hysterectomy. It will speed your recovery, improve your mood, and reduce the risk of weight gain. It reduces the number of hot flashes and increases blood flow to the brain. It also helps to keep your bones strong and definitely improves the health of your heart.

The best kind of exercise is weight-bearing exercise such as walking, aerobics, running, and sports. Studies have shown that to increase the mineral content of your bones, you need to exercise at least 30 minutes per day for 3 days per week. This equates to a *fast* 1.5-mile walk each day. Slow walking or swimming by itself is not sufficient. Muscle-building exercises also help you to maintain a "young" metabolism and avoid weight gain.

To stay motivated, choose a type of exercise that you enjoy. If you're walking, make a regular date with a companion or listen to music.

"I started doing Aquaform because I found that after the hysterectomy I gained quite a bit of weight, I'm not sure why—I suppose I sat around a lot and I wasn't too active, either."

Silvia

Smoking and Drinking

Apart from risking lung cancer and heart disease, women who smoke become menopausal earlier. Smoking also increases the risk of osteoporosis by leaching minerals from your bones. It is never too late (or too early) to stop smoking. Once you stop, your risks decrease dramatically. There are lots of ways to help you give up. Talk to your physician or a local support group.

For those who consume alcohol, moderation is the key. Alcohol is very high in calories, so it contributes to weight gain (rapidly). It also increases the risk of osteoporosis. For a while after your surgery, avoid it altogether as it may interact with your pain medication.

Caffeine has also been linked to osteoporosis, so you should also try to cut down on coffee, tea, and soft drinks that are high in caffeine if you are post-menopausal (check the label). Soft drinks can also irritate the bladder and are full of empty calories so you should try to avoid them as much as possible.

Weight Gain

Although it's a myth that hysterectomy causes weight gain by itself, you may be sitting around a little more after your operation, and no doubt indulging in a few extra treats, so it's easy to see how the

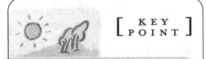

[**KEY POINT**]

Weight gain after hysterectomy (or menopause) is not inevitable. We know it's easier said than done, but the same rules still apply: burn more calories through exercise and eat fewer calories and you will lose weight.

pounds build up. Menopause, too, appears to result in more rapid weight gain, possibly due to a reduction in the metabolic rate. This is all bad news in many ways. Not only is it unhealthy for your heart, and leads to other health risks such as stroke or diabetes, but it will affect your self-image at a time when you need to feel great about yourself.

Unfortunately, there are only two reliable ways to lose weight: eating fewer calories (dieting) or burning more calories (exercising).

A combination of the two is even better. A gradual loss in weight usually works better than a sudden weight loss due to a crash diet. If you avoid fatty food and eat a balanced diet with lots of fruit and vegetables, and exercise on a regular basis, this may be all that you need to shed the extra pounds. Other good tips are: eating only I serving (or half the plate), avoiding snacks between meals, and cutting down on alcohol. Your doctor, a dietitian, or a support group can also help.

> "I was bad for the first 2 or 3 months, but after it's done, you shouldn't regret it, but tell yourself it was done, there was a reason for it, and you have to accept it, try to cope—and that takes time. With time, it heals."
>
> **Silvia**

Stress Management

Every life change involves large amounts of stress, which may go unrecognized for weeks, months, or even years. Some of us cope with stress better than others, but there is no doubt that you have the perfect excuse for feeling stressed after major surgery—especially if you are also coping with menopause.

The good news is that stress management is now a major industry in North America. This means that there are lots of good suggestions out there for dealing with it, from formal disciplines such as yoga and Tai Chi to therapies such as massage. Sometimes all it takes is a really good relaxation technique. Some ideas are included below.

Deep Breathing and Relaxation

Learning to relax by deep breathing is a useful skill. Regular relaxation can reduce your blood pressure and pain and reduce the number of hot flashes. It also helps you feel more in control—especially useful during those undignified gynecological examinations. There are many different relaxation techniques and lots of tapes available to help you find one that suits you. The simplest is deep breathing. Find a quiet place where you are unlikely to be interrupted and sit or lie comfortably. Take slow, deep breaths through your nose and as you breathe out, repeat a comforting word or phrase to yourself, such as "my health matters."

Tai Chi and Yoga

Tai Chi is a form of exercise that involves slow, controlled arm movements with weight regularly shifted from one leg to another. Not only is this helpful in reducing stress, it improves balance and can reduce falls in elderly people. Yoga strengthens muscles and increases flexibility, and is another excellent stress-reducer. Many neighborhoods offer yoga and Tai Chi classes.

Massage

Massage is the art of using the hands to stimulate the skin and muscles to bring about a feeling of comfort and to promote healing. There are many forms of massage, including Swedish, shiatsu, aromatherapy, reflexology, and neuromuscular. It can be a very positive experience and is the perfect way to reduce stress.

> "You need to pamper yourself, too. I booked myself a nice facial for an hour and I also went out and bought new, comfortable pants."
>
> **Silvia**

Other Complementary Therapies

Visualization

This is a form of meditation that involves using mental imagery to bring about the changes that you wish for. The idea—a visual version of "positive thinking," which may explain its apparent success in some people—is to believe that the more clearly you can see your desired future, the more chances there are of it becoming true. Many people find that visualization works well for surgery. You could visualize your procedure and welcome it in a positive way, seeing it as a means to an end, a necessary part of the healing process. It works best if you divide the images into the different stages of your procedure, such as, going to the hospital, getting ready, the procedure itself, returning to the hospital room and returning to your regular life. You can now buy tapes to help you with pre-surgery visualization (see Resources).

Acupuncture

Acupuncture has been in use in China for over 3,500 years and involves inserting fine needles into the skin and underlying tissues. Acupuncture practitioners consider acupuncture to work by stimulating the person's "vital force" or *qi* (pronounced chee). Although science has neither proven nor disproven that acupuncture works this way, we do know that it is helpful for pain, nausea and vomiting. It is not clear whether it works for menopausal symptoms.

Herbal Remedies

Herbs have been used as medicines since the beginning of humankind, and many of today's prescription medicines are based on natural substances found in herbs. Although there are numerous herbs suggested for use in healing and menopause, not all of them have been tested scientifically, so maintain a healthy skepticism of extravagant claims. However, many have well-documented effects and these are covered below.

Warning: If you are considering the use of herbs, we strongly advise that you consult an experienced herbalist or naturopathic doctor. Herbs and prescription drugs can interact, with serious side effects.

Pre-Surgery

Echinacea is well-known for its immune-boosting abilities. It can be taken up to 1 week prior to surgery and continued for 7 to 10 days afterward to help healing. Echinacea has no known adverse effects, but short-term use is advised. If you are taking immunosuppressive drugs, get some advice before taking echinacea.

Post-Surgery

Chamomile is a very gentle healing herb with antimicrobial and anti-inflammatory properties. As an oil, it can be rubbed on your abdominal area after surgery, but avoid your actual wounds until they have healed over. **Fennel tea** is a great way to alleviate digestive problems after surgery. For constipation, avoid herbal laxatives, which can be addictive, and simply try adding more liquid, oats, or stewed apple to your diet.

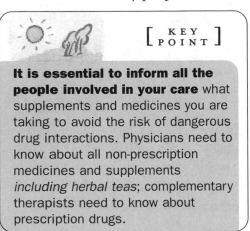

[KEY POINT]

It is essential to inform all the people involved in your care what supplements and medicines you are taking to avoid the risk of dangerous drug interactions. Physicians need to know about all non-prescription medicines and supplements *including herbal teas*; complementary therapists need to know about prescription drugs.

Herbs for Menopause

There are numerous herbs that have been proven effective for the symptoms of menopause, although their effects on the long-term risks such as osteoporosis or heart disease are still unknown.

Chasteberry

This herb has been used for centuries for "women's complaints." The berries are used either fresh, dry, or as a liquid extract. In one large study published in a recent edition of the *British Medical Journal*, **chasteberry** reduced premenstrual symptoms by 50 percent overall, including irritability, mood alteration, anger, headache, breast fullness, and bloating.

Ginkgo

Ginkgo has been shown to relieve premenstrual symptoms in women approaching menopause. This includes improvements in breast tenderness, bloating, anxiety, depression, and headaches. However, it does reduce blood clotting so stop using it at least 2 weeks before your surgery and don't take it with other blood thinners such as warfarin (e.g., Coumadin).

Phytoestrogens

Phytoestrogens are mild estrogens found in plants. There are three different types: **isoflavones**, **lignins**, and **coumestans**. They may help with menopausal symptoms such as hot flashes and there is also some evidence that diets high in phytoestrogens (such as soy, see below) reduce the risk of heart disease. They are found in more than 300 plant foods, including parsley, garlic, grains (wheat, rice, and soybeans), fruits (dates, cherries and apples), coffee, and wine. Asian diets are rich in isoflavones (40 to 80 mg daily), whereas Western diets contain less than 3 mg of isoflavones daily.

Black Cohosh

This native North American herb is probably the most effective phytoestrogen. Several clinical studies have shown that it can calm hot flashes, reduce night sweats, help relieve menstrual pain, relieve headaches, and ease joint pain. It has also been shown to reduce blood pressure and improve circulation. It should not be taken for longer than 6 months and avoided in women with menstrual "flooding." Side effects may include frontal headaches and stomach complaints. An overdose can result in vertigo, visual disturbance, nausea, and vomiting. Do not use it in combination with hormonal replacement therapy (HRT) as this may decrease the effectiveness of both treatments.

There has been much discussion recently as to whether **black cohosh** is suitable for women who have breast cancer. The bottom line is that women with breast cancer may want to avoid black cohosh until its effects on breast tissue are understood.

Red Clover

Red clover contains phytoestrogens and has been receiving increasing attention as a treatment for menopausal symptoms such as hot flashes and anxiety. However, there is a lack of scientific evidence confirming that red clover is truly effective for menopausal symptoms.

Wild or Mexican Yam

Despite recent excitement over these "natural hormone" products, there is no evidence that these creams actually work. The manufacturers obviously have the same concern because, according to the American College of Obstetrics and Gynecology, some Mexican yam products are boosted with artificial progesterone, and many contain no estrogen at all. The advice here is to save your money and spend it elsewhere.

Soy

   Soy is high in isoflavones, a type of phytoestrogen. It can lower "bad" cholesterol levels and appears to have an effect on menopausal symptoms such as hot flashes and vaginal dryness. However, because soy acts like an estrogen, it will cause thickening of the uterine lining, so reduce your soy intake if you still have bleeding problems. Women with breast cancer should also avoid it. Integrating soy into your diet is probably more beneficial than taking soy supplements.

Caution with the Complementaries

[**MORE DETAIL**]

Just because a herb or supplement is "natural" doesn't mean it's safe—the natural world contains some of our most powerful poisons. Herbs will act like drugs in the body, with bad effects as well as good effects. Plant estrogens, for example, will thicken the lining of the uterus and may be dangerous for women with breast cancer. They also have the potential to interfere with other medicines.

Remember, too, that herbal treatments are not as well researched as conventional medicines, which have to undergo years of trials in humans so that we know all about the side effects and which patients they are best for. Complementary therapies don't have to jump through these hoops, so be wary of over-optimistic claims, especially if they are based on "testimonials." This is usually a sure sign that no science-based studies exist.

Finally, be aware that complementary therapies may have hidden ingredients that are not declared on labeling. So-called natural hormone creams are often laced with artificial hormones to make them more effective. Many pills have added caffeine for a quick "pick-me-up."

If you are thinking of taking herbs or other supplements, consult a qualified herbalist or naturopath or mention them to your physician so that he or she can check out any downsides.

Your Sex Life

As we discussed in Chapter 9, *in general* hysterectomy makes little or no difference to a woman's sex life, and, in fact, many women enjoy sex more because they no longer have to worry about bleeding, discomfort, or the fear of becoming pregnant. However, everyone's experience is different so if you are disappointed or struggling, some of the suggestions below may help. Also, do not be afraid to talk to your physician. If you don't get the answers you need, ask to be referred to someone who specializes in sexual difficulties.

"I'm not sure why some people have more difficulty achieving orgasm after a hysterectomy. Your main erotic stimulus is your clitoris and you've done nothing to that. There's probably a whole bunch of things, not just the surgery."

Dawn

The Power of the Mind

Remember that the brain is the most powerful sex organ of all. If you tell yourself that hysterectomy will affect your orgasm, it probably will. Conversely, read Chapter 9 again and tell yourself that there is absolutely no anatomical reason why you should not orgasm the same as before and see what happens.

Remember, too, that time is the great healer. You may still be tired and unwell from your procedure, so tell yourself that your sex life will improve once you feel better.

You can also provide your brain with some raw material to work on. Try putting yourself "in the mood" with erotic books or videos, or buying some new silky underwear. Also, don't underestimate the power of love and tenderness. Set aside time for you and your partner to be together. Go out for meals, take a long walk together—or a long weekend—and just enjoy each other's company again without the pressure of sex.

Kegel Exercises

The aim of Kegel exercises is to strengthen the muscles that support and surround the vagina (see More Detail box on page 168). When done regularly, they not only help with medical problems such as urinary incontinence or vaginal prolapse, but can improve sex by allowing the vagina to grip the penis more strongly. It is probably best not to start them until about a week after surgery.

Vaginal Lubrication

Vaginal lubrication is controlled by estrogen, so you may find that your vagina feels drier after menopause and that you don't lubricate as fast during sex. This is not a sign that you are "less interested", it's just a physiological fact of life. Fortunately, there is plenty you can do about it. Estrogen replacement therapy (Chapter 12) will help a lot. If you don't want to take tablets, estrogen cream for your vagina can help, although you should avoid using this just before sex as it may be absorbed by your partner's penis. Vaginal lubricants are also helpful. The simplest is probably saliva, although some couples find that water-soluble lubricants like K-Y Jelly work well. Don't use Vaseline or other petroleum-based products as a lubricant as they can damage condoms and irritate sensitive tissues. Be sure to avoid washing the vulva with soap. Antibacterial, scented, and even so-called "moisturizing" soaps can be drying and irritating, making sex uncomfortable or even painful. Vaginal lubrication can also be improved in some women by a medical device available on prescription from your physician called **Eros**, which applies gentle suction to the clitoris.

Kegel Exercises

These simple exercises were invented by a gynecologist named Arnold Kegel to treat urinary incontinence. They may also help improve your sex life. They will be familiar to women who have had children, but a refresher course won't hurt. The great part about Kegels is that you can do them anywhere—on the subway, standing in a grocery store line, or watching TV.

1. Lie on your back with your knees bent. Contract and hold your vaginal muscles for a count of 4 by imagining that you are holding a tampon in place. Relax for 10 seconds. Remember to breathe while you are holding the contraction.

2. Do this 5 times, 3 times a day for a couple of weeks.

3. When you can do this without problems, try "the flutter." This involves contracting and relaxing rapidly, without a rest in-between.

4. Try both types of exercises in different positions, such as sitting or standing up.

5. Next, try the "drawing-in" exercise. This involves imagining that you are slowly drawing something right up inside you. Do 5 repetitions, 3 times a day.

6. Repeat all these exercises several times a day.

Increase Stimulation

Unless you're going it alone, you'll have to involve your partner in this suggestion. Remember that after menopause there is reduced blood flow to your vagina and clitoris so they may need more stimulation to reach orgasm. Again, this is not a sign that something is "wrong with you," it's just physiology. Explore ways to increase your stimulation, such as a longer period of foreplay, the use of a vibrator, or more clitoral stimulation than before. You can also try to find your "G-spot," if you have not already done so (page 6). It is also worth knowing that regular exercise increases blood flow to the vagina and vulva and may therefore help to improve sensation.

Simple Pleasuring

If sex is becoming an issue and things are getting tense in the bedroom, try taking a step back and re-discovering the pleasure of each other's bodies without worrying about orgasms. Sex need not follow the same step-by-step route to orgasm each time. Start slowly with no particular goals in mind. Hugging and kissing are just fine without always moving on to sex. A full-body massage, or just a foot massage, feels absolutely wonderful from a loving partner. Once both of you have re-learned to love the journey as well as the destination, you may have no problem finding your way.

Help Yourself to a Healthy Future

- Make sure you have a complete medical examination, gynecological examination, and breast examination annually.
- Have a mammogram every 1-2 years if you are over 40, and yearly after you reach 50
- Do breast self-examination regularly
- Give up smoking
- Exercise regularly
- Drink alcohol sparingly
- Control your weight
- Eat a healthy, calcium-rich diet and restrict your intake of caffeine
- Manage stress by breathing or relaxation exercises, yoga, Tai Chi, or meditation
- Get plenty of sleep.

Breast Self-Examination

Most women believe in the importance of breast self-examination, but they don't do it regularly or only for a few months—usually after a doctor's visit. Then they forget about it until they are reminded again by their physician or when they learn about a friend or relative who is diagnosed with breast cancer. The best time to examine your breasts is after your menstrual period, but any time is a good time and it should be done every month. After hysterectomy it is easiest to do your exam on the first day of each month.

- First, stand normally with your arms relaxed at your sides in front of a mirror with good lighting and look at the overall appearance of your breasts. Look for any changes in the shape and size of your breasts, or the skin's appearance.

- Raise both arms over your head and see whether your breasts move up and down together and check the appearance of your breasts again.

- Use your right hand to examine your left breast with your left hand relaxed at your side. Then use your left hand to examine your right breast with your right hand relaxed at your side. Move the pads of your fingers slowly in a small circular motion (like rolling dough) and rotate your fingers around the breast. If you feel a lump or hard tissue, contact your physician and he or she will recheck it. Note that the tail of your breast is located under your armpit.

- Repeat the examination with one hand behind your head.

- Do it again with one hand on your waist.

- Then repeat the same motions when you are lying on your back.

- Check for discharge from your nipples. If there is a bloody discharge, see your physician right away.

This may sound complicated, but it will only take a few minutes of your time each month.

What Happens Next?

Now that you are fully equipped to enjoy your new life, go ahead and enjoy it. Don't forget your annual checkups and remember to tell your physician about any complementary treatments that you undertake.

Chapter 11

has my hysterectomy worked?

What Happens in this Chapter

- What you might expect right away
- The long-term picture
- Likely results for pelvic pain and endometriosis
- Post-surgical problems

Unless you had a hysterectomy to treat life-threatening bleeding or cancer, the result you are looking for is simply an improvement in your quality of life. Women with heavy bleeding, fibroids, or prolapse should immediately feel benefits. Endometriosis or chronic pelvic pain may need additional treatment if surgery has not provided the cure. Post-surgery complications may also affect how pleased you are with the results of your surgery.

Immediate Results

IMMEDIATELY AFTER YOUR HYSTERECTOMY YOUR GYNECOLOGIC surgeon will speak to your relatives or friends and let them know that all is well. Once you are awake, he or she will also talk to you and discuss whether the procedure went as planned. If you had a hysterectomy for cancer or suspected cancer, you won't know the results of the laboratory tests for about 2 weeks, by which point you will be at home, so call your doctor's office for your results. Knowing that you do not have cancer, or that the cancer has been completely removed, will give you a sense of relief.

The Long-Term Picture

The purpose of hysterectomy is to improve your quality of life. So how can you tell if life has improved?

What You Might Expect

- You will not have periods anymore and your menstrual pain will disappear. You will feel better and stronger, and your blood-iron levels will gradually increase.

- If you had large fibroids, your abdomen will be smaller and you will need to urinate less frequently.

- If you had endometriosis, your pain should diminish or disappear, especially if you had your ovaries removed.

- If you had a sagging uterus (prolapse), there will be no more sensations of pressure and you may be in less pain.

- If you had early cancer confined to the uterus, this will be gone and you will not have to undergo further treatment with chemotherapy or radiation. Nevertheless, a close follow-up by your gynecologist is crucial, so don't forget your appointments.

What If There's No Change?

Although studies show that the vast majority of women are happy with the results of their hysterectomy, around 1 in 10 finds no change in their symptoms. This is much more likely if you had hysterectomy for chronic (long-term) pelvic pain or endometriosis, especially if your ovaries were left in.

> "I think women have to be given credit for their own intelligence. They need to listen to advice, but then I think they should go with their feelings. For the first few days they'll definitely know they had surgery, but they're going to be fine. My advice is to hold on, get a couple of good books and enjoy the rest, because life is going to come at you again full force and you'll feel better than ever."
>
> **Anne**

Chronic Pelvic Pain

If you had a hysterectomy for chronic pelvic pain and it is not cured, it is likely that the pain was caused by something else, possibly an intestinal or urinary problem, chronic muscle tension, or stress. Get help from your physician, who may suggest a checkup by a specialist in these areas. You may also be in discomfort because of a post-surgical problem, described below. Sometimes no specific cause is found. Stress control, biofeedback, acupuncture, relaxation training, or counseling can be very effective.

Endometriosis

Hysterectomy cures endometriosis pain in many women, but not all, which is one of the reasons why many gynecologists are reluctant to do hysterectomy for endometriosis. A cure is more likely if the ovaries are removed as well. In a large study that followed women for 5 years after hysterectomy for endometriosis, symptoms returned in 6 out of 10 women whose ovaries were left in, and about half of these needed more surgery. By contrast, symptoms came back in only 1 in 10 of those whose ovaries were removed. About one-third of these women went on to have more surgery.

Post-Surgical Problems

Several studies from around the world have shown that the medical problems after surgery are the most common reason that women are dissatisfied with their hysterectomy.

A rare but serious medical complication is intestinal blockage from **adhesions**, fibrous curtains of scar tissue that form after any operation, connecting two or more organs. Intestinal blockage after abdominal hysterectomy happens in about 4 in 1,000 women within a few years of surgery. It is very rare after vaginal or laparoscopic hysterectomy.

If this happens to you, you will feel sick and dehydrated. You will vomit, be unable to have a bowel movement or pass gas, and your abdomen will swell. If you experience these symptoms within a few years of your hysterectomy, contact your doctor or go to the emergency room. In some cases, the blockage opens by itself. If it doesn't, surgery is needed to release it.

[KEY POINT]

Intestinal blockage is a rare, but serious, consequence of hysterectomy that can develop years after your surgery. Symptoms are vomiting, severe constipation, abdominal swelling, and dehydration. Get medical help right away.

Emotional problems after surgery may also interfere with quality of life after surgery. However, as discussed elsewhere (page 150), studies show that hysterectomy itself does not "cause" depression. Other factors are usually at play, including fear of aging, fatigue, or the "empty nest" syndrome.

Sexual difficulties are also a potential complication, although, as we discussed at length in other parts of this book (pages 145 to 150), they are the exception rather than the rule.

> "For me what happened wasn't fair, but the decision was right. I had done almost everything I could to save my uterus and to be healthy, but as much as I tried hormone treatments, birth control pills, and laparoscopies to find out what was wrong, I suffered for that. If I knew then what I know now, I think I would have done it even earlier."
>
> **Silvia**

What Happens Next?

In the vast majority of women, hysterectomy brings welcome relief. If you are still in pain, or experience any post-surgical problems, do not hesitate to go back to your physician. If all is well, simply enjoy a new, healthy life, and don't forget those annual checkups with your physician.

hormone replacement therapy

What Happens in this Chapter

- Hormone replacement therapy after a hysterectomy
- Benefits and side effects
- Skin patches, gels, rings, and creams
- Who should not take hormone therapy

If your ovaries were removed during your hysterectomy, you will immediately enter menopause. In this case, your physician will strongly suggest that you start taking estrogen replacement therapy (ERT) to avoid the short-term symptoms of menopause such as hot flashes and the long-term health risks, such as osteoporosis. You may also be prescribed other hormones, such as progesterone or testosterone.

Why Is HRT Necessary?

AS WE DISCUSSED IN CHAPTER 1, THE OVARIES PRODUCE THE SEX hormones estrogen and progesterone, and androgens such as testosterone, which affect in powerful ways how the body works. After the removal of both ovaries you will enter surgical menopause and have symptoms related to the absence of these hormones, such as hot flashes. The treatment, in which a medicine is used to replace these hormones, is called hormonal replacement therapy or HRT. In the past, estrogen only was used (**estrogen replacement therapy** or **ERT**). This was mainly to prevent hot flashes, but physicians soon realized that long-term estrogen therapy alone thickened the endometrium (lining of the uterus) and increased the risk of endometrial cancer. By adding artificial progesterone (**progestin**), this risk is averted.

If you have had a total hysterectomy, you will not need a progestin because you no longer have an endometrium. However, if you have a history of endometriosis or your cervix is still in place, adding a progestin may be a good idea because estrogen alone may stimulate any remaining endometrial tissue inside you.

Hormone replacement therapy is a controversial area and every week, it seems, a new study comes out with different findings. The great strength of estrogen is that it is very effective for the short-term symptoms of menopause, and protects bones against the long-term risk of osteoporosis. The big question mark concerns HRT's effects on heart disease and breast cancer. We now suspect that long-term use of ERT might be associated with a slight increase in breast cancer, and combined estrogen and progestin (i.e., HRT) may increase the risk of heart disease. Because of this, most physicians will prescribe hormones to relieve menopausal symptoms for as short a time period as possible.

The Benefits of HRT

The benefits of HRT include the following:

- Fewer hot flashes and the associated sleep disturbance, irritability, mood problems, and headaches
- Prevention of bone loss (osteoporosis)
- Improved health of the vagina and the urinary system. The lining of the vagina, urethra, and bladder become thick and well-lubricated again, making intercourse less painful, and reducing frequent urination and urinary infections
- Androgens can increase the sense of well-being, positive mood, and, maybe, sexual desire
- Enhanced sexual arousal and lubrication

The Downsides of HRT

Breast Cancer

The risk of breast cancer with estrogen therapy is still debated. Some large, impressive studies show there is no additional risk; other large, impressive studies show that there is. Bearing in mind that every woman has a 1 in 8 chance of getting breast cancer in her lifetime, the additional risk posed by ERT, if any, is likely to be small. However, if you are at higher than usual risk of breast cancer, for example if you have had it already, it is probably safer to avoid ERT. If your hysterectomy was done for endometrial cancer, you should also talk to your gynecologist about the wisdom of estrogen replacement.

Just in case, if you are taking ERT you should do a breast

self-exam every month without fail (see page 170) and have a mammogram every 1 to 2 years if you are in your forties and every year if you are over 50.

Thrombosis

There is good evidence that estrogen therapy increases the risk of blood clot formation in veins—a condition called **deep vein thrombosis** or DVT. However, the risk remains small: DVT occurs in approximately 3 out of every 10,000 women on ERT.

Heart Disease

Early studies on estrogen replacement therapy apparently indicated that it decreased the risk of heart disease. The problem is that the women who were taking estrogen in these studies were also more health-conscious generally, so the results were misleading. A recent, better-designed study showed that combination estrogen plus progesterone actually *increases* the risk of heart disease very slightly.

Other Side Effects

A lesser known downside of HRT is that it carries three times the risk of gallbladder disease (**gallstones**). And although there is no evidence that HRT causes weight gain, progestins, especially **medroxyprogesterone**, can make you feel heavier due to bloating or fluid retention. Fluid retention may also make existing conditions worse, such as epilepsy, asthma, heart disease, migraines, or kidney disease. Fluid retention is less of a problem with the progestin norethindrone. Progestins can also cause breast tenderness and low mood.

How Do You Take HRT?

Beside tablets taken by mouth, hormone therapy can also be given through the skin (patch and gel) or in the form of a vaginal suppository (vaginal ring). The hormone is absorbed through the skin or vaginal wall and enters the circulation directly, bypassing the stomach and liver. The result is a nearly constant level of hormones in the blood. The table on page 185 shows some common types of HRT.

Skin Patches

As their name implies, **estrogen patches** are sticky patches saturated with medication. They should be applied on clean and dry skin that is not exposed to the sun. The best sites are the buttocks or lower abdomen. Avoid the breast area because of the potentially dangerous effects of estrogen on breast tissue. Most patches are changed twice a week. They are very convenient, but about 7 in 100 women discontinue the patch due to skin irritation.

Estrogen Gel

Estrogen gel is a colorless, odorless gel designed to be applied daily to a large area of the skin, usually the arms. The abdomen or inner thigh are also good places. Because estrogen has beneficial effects on skin collagen, some women apply estrogen gel to their faces to prevent wrinkling. While studies show that this does work to some extent, be warned that estrogen also increases blood flow, so your face will become flushed.

Estrogen Ring

The estrogen ring is inserted into the upper vagina for up to 3 months. Although it can slide out of the vagina, especially if you have a prolapsed uterus or vagina, most women tolerate it fairly well. The most common reasons for discontinuing the ring are vaginal irritation and nausea.

Vaginal Cream

Estrogen cream is mainly used to treat painful intercourse due to a dry vagina. The hormone works on the spot to increase the thickness of the vaginal wall and improve vaginal lubrication. Although some is absorbed into the circulation, the level is usually too low to relieve other symptoms such as hot flashes, or to prevent osteoporosis.

Types of HRT

There are many different HRT regimes, and your physician will discuss with you the one that he or she thinks will suit you best.

Estrogen and Progestin

Continuous estrogen is for women who have had a hysterectomy and have no history of endometriosis. Examples are: 0.625 mg of Premarin or 1 mg of Estrace per day.

Progestin-only pills are for women who cannot take estrogen, but suffer from hot flashes.

Cyclic estrogen and progestin regimes take many forms; their aim is to add some progestin, but not too much, to keep progestin side effects to a minimum. Examples include: continuous use of FemPatch or an Estraderm patch from days 1 to 25 plus Provera or Prometrium daily from days 14 to 25. The progestin is there to prevent reactivation of endometriosis. It is also recommended for those who have had a subtotal hysterectomy.

Continuous estrogen and progestin regimes may be even more effective for women with previous endometriosis or a subtotal hysterectomy. They are also the treatment of choice for women with an intact uterus. Here, both estrogen and progestin are given every day, for example Premarin or Estrace plus Provera or Prometrium daily (see table on page 185).

Androgens

Some HRT formulations also contain the "male" hormone testosterone (see page 12). Testosterone is normally made in small amounts by the ovaries, so levels will drop if you have your ovaries removed. When added to HRT, testosterone can be helpful for improving mood and libido, but be warned that it can also increase weight gain, acne, and facial hair growth. You may receive injections of an estrogen/testosterone combination in the hospital immediately after your surgery to tame severe hot flashes in the first few days.

What's in a Name? [**MORE DETAIL**]

Every drug has both a generic and a brand name. The generic name usually refers to the chemical structure of a drug and always stays the same, whereas the brand name can change over time, or differ in different countries.

Hormone Replacement Therapies

The brand names and generic names of some common types of HRT are shown below, along with their doses.

Brand name	Generic name
Estrogen Tablets	
Premarin	conjugated estrogen
Estrace	estradiol-17ß
Ogen	estropipate
Ortho-Est	estropipate
Estrogen Patches	
Climara	estradiol-17ß
Vivelle-Dot	estradiol-17ß
Estraderm	estradiol-17ß
FemPatch	estradiol-17ß
Estrogen Gel	
Estrogel	estradiol-17ß hemihydrate
Estrogen Insert	
Estring	estradiol-17ß
Femring	estradiol-17ß
Progestin Tablets	
Provera	medroxyprogesterone acetate
Prometrium	progesterone (12 days)
Aygestin	norethindrone
Combined Estrogen-Progestin Tablets	
Activella	estradiol-17ß + norethindrone acetate
Ortho-Prefest	estradiol-17ß (days 1-6) + norgestimate (days 4-6), then repeat cycle
PremPhase	conjugated estrogen (28 days) + medroxyprogesterone acetate (14 days)
Prempro	conjugated estrogen + medroxyprogesterone acetate
FemHRT	ethinyl estradiol + norethindrone
Combined Estrogen-Progestin Patches	
CombiPatch	estradiol-17ß (28 days) + norethindrone acetate (14 days)
Combined Estrogen-Testosterone Injection	
Depo-Testadial	testosterone cypionate + estradiol cypionate
Combined Estrogen-Testosterone Pill	
Estratest	esterified estrogen + methyltestosterone

Designer Drugs

Because estrogen stimulates the uterine lining and breast tissue to grow and potentially turn cancerous, researchers continue searching for better non-estrogen drugs to treat post-menopausal women. The drug raloxifene (Evista) was designed with this in mind. This **selective estrogen receptor modulator (SERM)** is not an estrogen and cannot treat the short-term symptoms of menopause like hot flashes (in fact, hot flashes are one of its side effects), but it does provide protection against osteoporosis and reduce blood cholesterol without stimulating the uterine lining. Like its sister drug tamoxifen, Evista also seems to decrease the risk of breast cancer.

An interesting experimental drug called tibolone may also provide a solution. Although not yet approved for use in North America, it appears to promise the best of all possible worlds. Studies show that it seems to act as a combination of estrogen, progestin, and testosterone, decreasing hot flashes and protecting bones without thickening the uterine lining. Like estrogen, it also improves vaginal dryness and makes intercourse less painful. Whether this promise will be fulfilled remains to be seen once all the studies are complete.

[**KEY POINT**]

You should not take HRT if you have:

- unexplained vaginal bleeding
- active liver disease
- a personal history of breast cancer
- cancer of the uterus
- a history of blood clots in your legs (deep vein thrombosis) or lungs (pulmonary embolism)
- a very inactive lifestyle, for instance, due to a recent stroke, a hip fracture, or heart attack.

What Happens Next?

Hormone replacement therapy is just one part of ensuring your long-term health after menopause. Don't forget that a calcium-rich diet and plenty of exercise will also protect your bones and heart (see Chapter 10) and should go hand in hand with any medical therapy. Many women discontinue HRT after a year or so due to the fear of long-term risks, or unpleasant side effects. If you are considering doing so, talk to your physician before stopping your therapy yourself. He or she may be able to suggest an alternative that suits you better.

Chapter 13

future directions in hysterectomy

What Happens in this Chapter

- Clinical trials and you
- Trends in hysterectomy
- Fertility sparing and nerve-sparing techniques
- Future alternatives to hysterectomy

Hysterectomy has improved the lives of millions of women, but there is always room for improvement. Many exciting developments are underway, both in hysterectomy and the alternatives. Minimally invasive hysterectomy is becoming increasingly common, and researchers are finding better ways to spare the cervix, the pelvic nerves, and fertility. Better alternatives on the horizon include ultrasound destruction of fibroids without surgery and photodynamic therapy.

Clinical Trials and You

NEW TECHNIQUES AND INSTRUMENTS ARE CONTINUOUSLY INVENTED and perfected, but newer is not always better. In order to see whether they are as good or better than standard techniques, studies are needed.

If you are approached to participate in a clinical study, carefully read the documents the physician or research nurse gives you before agreeing to anything. If you want to take part, you will be asked to sign a consent form. If you want to know more about the study, ask, and if you are doubtful about participating, do not be afraid to say no. It is entirely your decision, and if you decide not to take part it will in no way affect the management of your condition. You can also withdraw from the study at any time without affecting your current or future treatment.

Trends in Hysterectomy

There is a general trend for surgery to be done through smaller and smaller incisions. This so-called minimally invasive surgery or laparoscopic surgery is now an option for hysterectomy, as this book shows. Laparoscopic surgery is much easier on patients than abdominal surgery because of the smaller cuts, reduced post-operative pain, faster recovery, and faster return to work. Until recently, laparoscopy tended to be reserved for non-cancerous, subtotal hysterectomies. As more surgeons train on the technique, we may see more radical hysterectomies being performed this way.

Another trend is the increase in the number of subtotal hysterectomies, where the cervix is left in place. This is now increasingly common in an effort to reduce damage to the ureter, the tube that runs from the kidney to the bladder. Surgeons also hope that this will minimize the effects on sexual function, although as yet there is no strong evidence either way that leaving the cervix makes any difference.

Advances in Cancer Treatment

The standard treatment for cancer of either the cervix or endometrium is total hysterectomy, with or without removal of both ovaries. In younger women who still want children this is a heart-breaking moment and techniques are being tested that will preserve the uterus until the woman's family is complete.

A regime of high-dose progestins is being tested in young women with early stage endometrial cancer. So far, some of the women have had children after this therapy, but the number of women treated is still limited and the potential for spread of the cancer is unknown. This treatment is definitely still in the "experimental" category.

In cervical cancer, a fertility-preserving technique that involves removal of the cervix only (**trachelectomy**) and the pelvic lymph nodes is being tried. If laboratory results during the procedure show that the cancer has not spread to the nodes, the surgeon will proceed with trachelectomy only. Otherwise, he or she will carry out a radical hysterectomy. If you want to explore this option, contact your doctor or ask for a second opinion.

Other New Techniques

Robotic surgery is entering the gynecological field, as everywhere else. There is no cause for alarm: a robot will not do the surgery, only remote-controlled robotic arms. In this experimental technique, the surgeon operates using two joysticks that are similar to the laparoscopic instruments, with the real instruments held in the abdomen by the robotic arms. The advantage of this technology is that the surgeon can operate from another city if necessary, a plus for remote communities, but it is unlikely to replace conventional laparoscopic hysterectomy.

A more promising technique is **nerve-sparing hysterectomy**. Radical hysterectomy carries a risk of damage to the pelvic nerves, causing impaired bladder function, defecation problems, and sexual dysfunction. Japanese researchers are perfecting a technique to preserve these nerves and the early results have been promising.

Hysterectomy Alternatives

Photodynamic Therapy

Many techniques are being developed for safer and more effective endometrial ablation (page 112). A new approach is **photodynamic therapy (PDT)**, currently used for throat cancer, in which a light-sensitive dye is injected into the uterus and stains the endometrium. A special light is then inserted into the uterus, which converts the dye into a toxic compound that triggers the cells of the endometrium to self-destruct. PDT is potentially useful for the treatment of endometriosis as well.

Fibroid Treatment Without Surgery

The only non-surgical treatment for fibroids currently available is uterine artery embolization (page 108). However, the risk that it will reduce fertility makes it unattractive to young women. Researchers are currently looking at ways to shrink fibroids by destroying them through the skin. One technique called **interstitial thermoablation** uses high-intensity ultrasound focused on the fibroid and so far it works in mice. If it proves to be effective, it will have huge advantages because the procedure does not require an incision and actually does not even need to enter the body, allowing for rapid healing.

Chapter 14

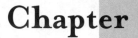

who's who of hospital staff

What Happens in this Chapter

- Hospital staff you will meet
- A brief description of their roles

When you go into the hospital, you will encounter a large number of staff. In general, they will be friendly and helpful. If you are dealing with them directly, they should introduce themselves and explain their role in your case.

However, many of the hospital staff, from porters to doctors wear a white coat or "scrubs" (loose pants and tops of all different colors), making it hard to figure out who's who. Also, within the title of "doctor" or "nurse" are a number of different roles, making it difficult to understand what each of these people do. For example, you may see a **fellow**, **a resident** or a **staff physician**. All are doctors, but they have varying levels of knowledge, ability, and responsibility. Or, you may see a **ward nurse**, a **recovery room nurse**, or a **research nurse**. Again, all are qualified nurses, but each has a different role.

This chapter will give you a brief overview, explaining who is who in the hospital and each person's role in your care.

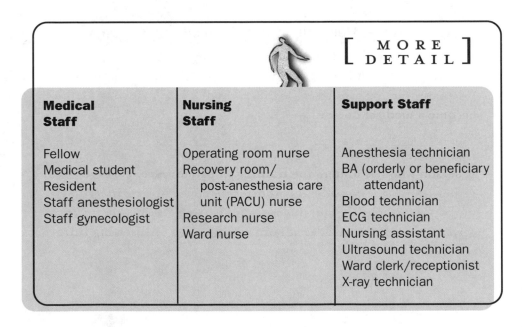

[**MORE DETAIL**]

Medical Staff	Nursing Staff	Support Staff
Fellow	Operating room nurse	Anesthesia technician
Medical student	Recovery room/	BA (orderly or beneficiary
Resident	post-anesthesia care	attendant)
Staff anesthesiologist	unit (PACU) nurse	Blood technician
Staff gynecologist	Research nurse	ECG technician
	Ward nurse	Nursing assistant
		Ultrasound technician
		Ward clerk/receptionist
		X-ray technician

Anesthesia Technician

A person who is trained to assist the anesthesiologist in caring for a patient while the patient is under anesthesia.

Blood Technician

A person who is specifically trained to take blood from patients, usually from the arm.

ECG Technician

A person who is specifically trained to perform ECGs on patients.

Fellow

A fully qualified doctor who has specialized training in a particular area of medicine or surgery, usually with a few years of experience. Fellows can come from other countries to spend up to 3 years gaining additional experience. For example, an obstetrician and gynecologist who wants to sub-specialize in reproductive endocrinology and infertility can apply for fellowship training that will last 2 to 3 years.

Medical Student

A person who is enrolled in medical school and is being trained to become a medical doctor.

Nursing Assistant

A person who has undergone training in patient care. However, his or her training is considerably shorter than that of a registered nurse. As a result, the nursing assistant is not permitted to perform certain procedures, such as administering drugs or inserting intra-venous lines.

Operating Room Nurse

A qualified nurse who works in the operating room. These nurses oversee and organize day-to-day surgery. They are responsible for the surgical instruments and they make sure that your needs are met before, during, and immediately after surgery. If you are feeling anxious right before your hysterectomy, the operating room nurse is a good person to talk to.

Orderly

A hospital attendant who works on the ward or the operating room under the direction of a nurse. An orderly will bring you to and from the operating room.

Recovery Room/PACU nurse

A qualified nurse who is responsible for patient care after transfer to the recovery room. The PACU nurse will make sure that your vital signs are stable and you receive adequate pain medication. He or she plays an important role in your care immediately after you wake up from anesthesia.

Research Nurse

A nurse who usually has a university degree and specializes in assisting and coordinating research. It is his or her job to approach patients for possible participation in research studies and co-ordinate their involvement in these studies. In some instances, the research nurse is also responsible for collecting blood samples for the studies and will see participants at follow-up appointments.

Resident

A licensed physician undergoing specialized training. He or she can specialize in a particular field, such as obstetrics and gynecology.

Staff Anesthesiologist

A doctor who administers anesthesia to reduce or eliminate pain and put surgery patients to sleep. The anesthesiologist's job includes medically evaluating patients before surgery, consulting with the surgical team, providing pain control, support of life during surgery, making decisions about blood conservation and transfusions, supervising care after surgery, and discharging patients from the recovery unit or intensive care unit.

Staff Gynecologist

An experienced doctor who has undergone formal training in obstetrics and gynecology. Some of these doctors have undergone sub-specialty or fellowship training in a more specific area of gynecology or obstetrics, such as advanced operative laparoscopy or high-risk pregnancy.

Ultrasound Technician

A person who is specifically trained to perform ultrasound on a patient. Ultrasound technicians who perform gynecological ultrasounds are usually female.

Ward Clerk/Receptionist

Usually the first person you will meet upon your arrival to the ward. He or she is responsible for organizing the administration of the ward. Often his or her role extends beyond this, depending on experience level.

Ward Nurse

A registered nurse (RN) who works on the ward providing patient care. Because these nurses work in shifts, you will encounter a few of them. They have a range of roles depending on seniority and experience and are responsible for your well-being and safety during your stay on the ward.

X-Ray Technician

A person who is specifically trained to take X-rays, or perform other imaging techniques. The X-ray technician may also assist with procedures such as uterine fibroid embolization.

Disclaimer: The above descriptions are intended as a general guide only. The roles of each type of staff member mentioned may differ slightly from hospital to hospital.

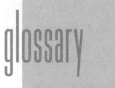

Acupuncture A complementary therapy that involves placing needles at specific points of the body to cure disease or relieve pain. Acupuncture originated in China and is now used worldwide.

Androgen A type of male hormone that can be found in small amounts in women, such as testosterone.

Anemia A deficiency in the number of red blood cells or in the amount of hemoglobin that the red blood cells contain.

Anesthetic A drug used to numb an area of skin ("local") or put someone to sleep ("general"). Hysterectomy is usually done under general anesthetic, which means you are completely asleep and will not feel any pain.

Anterior and posterior (AP) repair A procedure to re-position a sagging bladder or rectum.

Antibiotics Medicines used to treat bacterial infections.

Artery A blood vessel that carries oxygen-rich blood from the heart to the body tissues.

Atrophy The decrease in size of a body part, cell, organ, or tissue. Atrophy of the genitals is characterized by vaginal dryness and itch, and incontinence. This is due to a lack of estrogen after menopause.

Autologous blood donation Storing your own blood before surgery to be used after surgery in the event that you need a blood transfusion.

Catheter A narrow tube that is inserted into a part of the body.

Cautery An agent or tool used to burn tissue. In surgery, electrocautery (cautery using electric heat) is often used to seal blood vessels.

Cervix The lower, narrow part of the uterus that leads into the vagina.

Cholesterol A type of fat that accumulates in the walls of diseased blood vessels.

Clinical trial A study of a drug or procedure that involves patients.

Consent *See* Informed consent.

Dilation and curettage (D&C) A procedure to remove the inner lining of the uterus by scraping.

Dysfunctional uterine bleeding (DUB) Excessive bleeding from the uterus due to reduced ovulation.

ECG *See* Electrocardiogram.

Electrocardiogram (ECG) A record-ing of the electrical activity of your heart. An ECG takes just a few minutes and involves lying on a bed with a number of soft plastic electrodes stuck onto your body.

Electrocautery *See* Cautery.

Endometrial ablation A procedure in which the gynecologist destroys the lining of the uterus (endometrium) using electricity, heat, laser, microwave energy, or freezing.

Endometrial biopsy A small sample of the uterine lining, removed using a thin, plastic tube inserted into the uterus.

Endometrial cancer Cancer of the lining of the uterus.

Endometrial hyperplasia Thickening of the endometrium.

Endometriosis A condition in which cells like those in the uterus lining grow outside the uterus.

Endometrium The lining of the uterus.

Epidural anesthesia Injection of local anesthetic into the space surrounding the spinal canal, causing gradual numbness from the waist down.

Estrogen A sex hormone produced by the ovaries until menopause.

Factor XI deficiency A blood clotting disorder caused by deficiency of a substance needed for clotting.

Fallopian tubes Pairs of hollow tubes that extend from each side of the uterus to the ovaries. They allow sperm and eggs to pass from the ovaries to the uterus.

Femoral artery The artery in the groin. The catheter used in uterine fibroid embolization is inserted into the femoral artery.

Fibroid (myoma or leiomyoma) Harmless growths of muscle and fibrous tissue within the wall of the uterus. Submucous fibroids are fibroids located inside the uterus, just under the uterine lining. Intramural fibroids are located within the wall of the uterus. Subserous fibroids are on the outer surface of the uterus.

General anesthetic *See* Anesthetic.

Gynecology A medical specialty that deals with the female reproductive system.

Hemoglobin An iron-containing red pigment that is the main component of red blood cells, which deliver oxygen to the tissues. If you have an anemia, you do not have enough hemoglobin.

Herbal medicine Natural health product derived from plants that is classified as a food or dietary supplement, not a drug, e.g., ginseng and ginkgo biloba.

Hormone replacement therapy (HRT) Medicine containing estrogen, progesterone, or testosterone.

Hysterectomy Surgical removal of the uterus. Can be done via an incision in the abdomen or vagina, or by using a laparoscope.

Hysteroscopy Procedure in which a gynecologist uses a small telescopic instrument called a hysteroscope to check the inside of the uterus for abnormalities.

Incision A cut made during surgery.

Incontinence Inability of the body to control evacuative functions, such as urination (urinary incontinence).

Informed consent Consent that is obtained from a patient before he or she undergoes a medical procedure to diagnose or treat a condition.

Laparoscope A surgical telescope that allows a surgeon to look inside the abdomen and examine the internal organs, usually via a small incision below the navel.

Laparoscopy An operation using a laparoscope. The advantages of laparoscopic surgery are smaller incisions, less pain, and shorter recovery.

Laparotomy A surgical cut in the abdominal wall to gain entry into the abdomen.

Local anesthetic A drug that numbs the sensation of pain at the site of the injection.

Menopause The time when women stop menstruating and the ovaries stop functioning.

Menstruation (menses) The monthly shedding of the uterine lining that occurs if pregnancy does not occur; accompanied by vaginal bleeding.

Minimally invasive surgery Surgery that is performed using small or no incisions, for example vaginal and laparoscopic hysterectomy and hysteroscopic myomectomy.

Myolysis A technique for shrinking fibroids in which several deep holes are made inside a fibroid using a laser or long cautery needles.

Myomectomy An operation in which only the fibroids (or myomas) are removed, leaving the uterus intact.

Osteoporosis A disease characterized by the thinning of bones that break easily. Occurs most commonly after menopause due to a lack of estrogen.

Ovaries The main female reproductive organs that produce estrogen and progesterone. Equivalent to testes in males.

Papanicolau (Pap) test A test to detect cervical cancer or other abnormalities in the cervix.

Polyp A growth protruding from a mucous membrane. A polyp on the uterine lining is called an endometrial polyp.

Prolapse of the uterus A condition in which the uterus sinks down into the vagina due to weakness in its supporting structures.

Progestin Synthetic progesterone used in menopausal women to decrease their risk of endometrial cancer.

Regional anesthesia A type of anesthesia that blocks sensation to a particular region of the body by injecting anesthetic around the spinal nerves. *See also* Spinal anesthesia, Epidural anesthesia.

Saline instillation ultrasound An ultrasound examination that involves injecting a saline solution into the uterus. Good for detecting fibroids or polyps inside the uterus.

Scalpel A thin-bladed knife used in surgery.

Sedative A drug that lowers a patient's level of consciousness and makes him or her feel tired or sleepy. Sedatives can relax you if you are nervous before surgery.

Speculum examination Insertion of a metal or plastic instrument into the vagina so that the doctor can see the vagina and cervix. A speculum has two adjustable paddles that hold the vagina open.

Spinal anesthesia Injection of local anesthetic directly around the nerves of the spine causing rapid numbness from the waist down. *See also* Regional anesthesia.

Subtotal or supracervical hysterectomy Surgical removal of the uterus without removing the cervix.

Suture A stitch.

Total hysterectomy Surgical removal of the entire uterus including the cervix.

Transvaginal ultrasound Ultrasound using a probe inserted into the vagina.

Ultrasound An imaging technique that uses sound waves to create an image.

Uterine artery embolization *See* Uterine fibroid embolization.

Uterine fibroid embolization A procedure that shrinks fibroids by blocking the blood vessels of the uterus with tiny granules.

Uterus (womb) The pear-shaped, hollow organ in which a baby grows.

Vaginal hysterectomy Surgical removal of the uterus via the vagina.

Von Willebrand's disease A genetic bleeding disorder caused by a deficiency of a substance needed for blood clotting.

Hysterectomy Information

Hyster Sisters
2436 S. I-35 E. Suite 376-184
Denton, Texas 76205-4900
Hysterectomy recovery support.
http://www.hystersisters.com/05-4900

MEDLINEplus: Hysterectomy
Information on hysterectomy.
http://www.nlm.nih.gov/medlineplus/
hysterectomy.html

Centers for Disease Control and Prevention
Hysterectomy fact sheet.
http://www.cdc.gov/nccdphp/drh/
wh_hysterec.htm

New York State Info for Consumers
Information about the benefits, risks, and alternatives to hysterectomy.
http://www.health.state.ny.us/nysdoh/
consumer/women/hyster.htm

HERS Foundation
422 Bryn Mawr Avenue
Bala Cynwyd, PA 19004
Tel: (610) 667-7757
Toll Free: 1-888-750-HERS (1-888-750-4377)
Fax: (610) 667-8096
Email: info@hersfoundation.com
Information about hysterectomy, its adverse effects, and alternative treatments.
http://www.hersfoundation.com

OBGYN.net
P.O. Box 18297
Austin, TX 78760-8297
Tel: (512) 418-2922
Fax: (512) 339 9382
Physician-reviewed site offering medical professionals and women the latest news and information on hysterectomy and alternatives to hysterectomy.
http://www.obgyn.net/ah/ah.asp

Hysterectomy Support Society
Hysterectomy support group.
http://pub55.ezboard.com/bhysterectomysupportsociety

National Women's Health Network
514 10th St., N.W., Suite 400
Washington, DC 20004
(202) 628-7814
Information on hysterectomy and alternative techniques.
http://www.womenshealthnetwork.org

National Uterine Fibroids Foundation
1-877-553-NUFF (1-877-553-6833)
Information, research, and resources regarding uterine fibroids.
http://www.nuff.org

Endometriosis Association
1-800-992-3636
Information and support for women
with endometriosis.
http://www.endometriosisassn.org

Menopause Information

North American Menopause Society
Post Office Box 94527
Cleveland, OH 44101
Tel: (440) 442-7550
Toll Free: 1-800-774-5342
Fax: (440) 442-2660
Information and news about
menopause and therapies.
http://www.menopause.org/

Red Hot Mamas
23 North Valley Road
Ridgefield, Connecticut 06877
Tel: (203) 431-3902
Fax: (203) 894-1369
Menopause education and support
program.
http://www.redhotmamas.org

General Health Information

HealthFinder
A service of the U.S. Department of
Health and Human Services that
connects you to publications, non-
profit organizations, databases, web-
sites, and support groups.
http://www.healthfinder.gov

WebMD
Reliable health information including
news, disease and drug information,
health television guide, and tips for
making a personal health plan and for
searching the medical library.
http://www.webmd.com

**National Women's Health
Information Center**
1-800-994-WOMAN (1-800-994-
9662)
TDD (Telecommunications Device for
the Deaf): 1-888-220-5446
Information on women's health issues.
http://www.4woman.gov

Stress and Relaxation Information

**The Transcendental Meditation
Program**
Find out the benefits of, and how and
where to learn, transcendental
meditation.
http://www.tm.org

Meditation Society of America
Concepts and techniques of meditation
plus suggested reading.
http://www.meditationsociety.com

American Yoga Association
General information on yoga, how to
get started and how to choose a qualified yoga instructor.
http://www.americanyogaassociation.org

Nutrition and Fitness Information

American Dietetic Association
Daily tips and features about nutrition.
http://www.eatright.org

Books

Haas, Adelaide and Susan L. Puretz.
The Woman's Guide to Hysterectomy—
Expectations and Options. Revised Edition.
Celestial Arts, 2002.

Jones, Marcia L. and Theresa
Eichenwald. *Menopause for Dummies*.
Indianapolis. Wilcy Publishing, Inc.,
2003.

Rosenthal, M. Sara. *The Gynecological*
Sourcebook. Third Edition. Los Angeles:
Lowell House,1999.

Information on Alternative Therapies

Image Paths
891 Moe Drive, Suite C
Akron, Ohio 44310
Toll Free: 1-800-800-8661
Fax: (330) 633-3778
Visualization cassettes and CDs for
menopause and surgery.
http://www.healthjourneys.com

National Center for Complementary
and Alternative Medicine
Tel: (301) 231-7537, ext 5
Fax: (301) 495-4957
An official source of information,
including links to other sites, current
research, and scientific information.
http://www.nccam.nih.gov

Alternative Medicine Digest
What's new in alternative medicine.
http://www.alternativemedicine.com

MEDLINE Plus
Information on herbal remedies.
http://www.nlm.nih.gov/medlineplus/
herbalmedicine.html

National Center for Homeopathy
801 N. Fairfax Street, Suite 306
Alexandria, Virginia 22314
Tel: (703) 548-7790
Fax: (703) 548-7792
Homeopathic resources and research
information.
http://www.homeopathic.org

American Botanical Council
P.O. Box 144345
Austin TX 78714-4345
abc@herbalgram.org
Research, links, science-based
information on herbs and
phytomedicines.
http://www.herbalgram.org

Contact Information

Name of current family doctor:	Address:	Phone #:	Fax:	Email:
Hospital:	Address:	Phone #:	Fax:	Email:
Name of your gynecologist:	Address:	Phone #:	Fax:	Email:

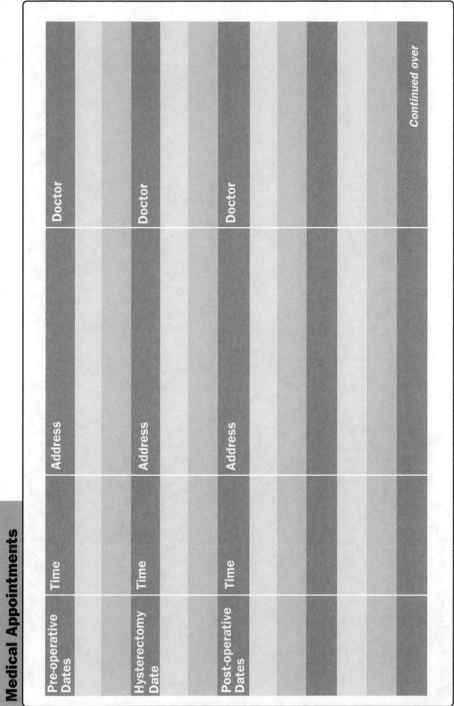

	Time	Address	Doctor
Pre-operative Dates			
Hysterectomy Date			
Post-operative Dates			

Continued over

Medical Appointments

Annual Checkup Date	Time	Address	Doctor
Mammogram Date	Time	Address	Doctor
Bone Density Date	Time	Address	Doctor

Current and Past Medications
(including complementary therapies and supplements)

Drug Name	Date Began Drug	Purpose of Drug	Dosage	Side Effects	Dosage Instructions

Current and Past Medications
(including complementary therapies and supplements)

Drug Name	Date Began Drug	Purpose of Drug	Dosage	Side Effects	Dosage Instructions

Symptoms

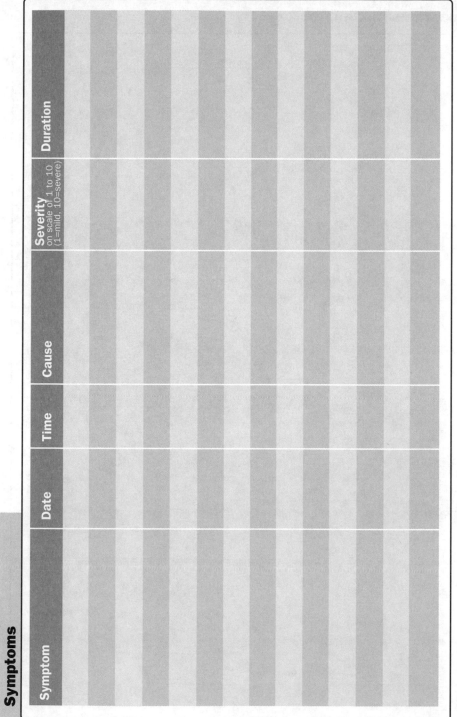

Symptom	Date	Time	Cause	Severity on scale of 1 to 10 (1=mild, 10=severe)	Duration

Questions for the Doctor

Contact Information

Wellness Center Contact Information

Address	Phone	Fax	Email

My Lifestyle Goals: Current Weight _____

Notes

Notes

index

References to figures: *3fig*;
references to tables: *119t*;
references to More Detail boxes in bold: **4**;
references to Key Point boxes in bold italic: ***5***;
references to Self-Help boxes in italic: *12*